WHAT I SAY

Conversations That Improve the Physician-Patient Relationship

WHAT I SAY

Conversations That Improve the Physician-Patient Relationship

Robert H. Osher, MD

Professor of Ophthalmology
University of Cincinnati College of Medicine
Medical Director Emeritus
Cincinnati Eye Institute
Cincinnati, Ohio
Editor
Video Journal of Cataract, Refractive, & Glaucoma Surgery
Program Director
Cataract Surgery: Telling It Like It Is! Meeting

Jack S. Parker, MD, PhD

Corneal Specialist
Parker Cornea
Birmingham, Alabama
Secretary and Director
The Netherlands Institute for Innovative Ocular Surgery USA

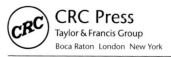

CRC Press
Taylor & Francis Group
Boca Raton   London   New York

CRC Press is an imprint of the
Taylor & Francis Group, an **informa** business

First published 2019 by SLACK Incorporated

Published 2024 by CRC Press
2385 NW Executive Center Drive, Suite 320, Boca Raton FL 33431

and by CRC Press
4 Park Square, Milton Park, Abingdon, Oxon, OX14 4RN

CRC Press is an imprint of Taylor & Francis Group, LLC

© 2019 Taylor & Francis Group, LLC

Library of Congress Cataloging-in-Publication Data

Names: Osher, Robert H., author. | Parker, Jack S., 1986- author.
Title: What I say : conversations that improve the physician-patient
    relationship / Robert H. Osher and Jack S. Parker.
Description: Thorofare, NJ : SLACK Incorporated, [2019] | Includes index.
Identifiers: LCCN 2019000235 (print) |ISBN 9781630916886 (pbk. : alk. paper)
Subjects: | MESH: Eye Diseases | Health Communication | Physician-Patient
    Relations | Ophthalmologic Surgical Procedures | Attitude of Health
    Personnel
Classification: LCC RE46 (print) | NLM WW 140 | DDC
    617.7--dc23
LC record available at https://lccn.loc.gov/2019000235

Cover Artist: Katherine Christie

ISBN: 9781630916886 (pbk)
ISBN: 9781003526926 (ebk)

DOI: 10.1201/9781003526926

Dedication

To our patients, our colleagues, our teachers,
and last but not least, our loving families.

CONTENTS

ACKNOWLEDGMENTS

This book is much more valuable because of the contributions from our invited roster of experts. Our thanks to each of you for sharing your difficult patient conversations. Others that deserve special thanks include Tonya Ragle and Linda Harris, who were indispensable in assembling and organizing the book's content.

As always, we also thank our families for the time and support necessary to complete these projects. Dr. Parker would like to thank his wife Christina, and Dr. Osher would like to acknowledge his parents Anne and Dr. Morris Osher (also an ophthalmologist), who together instilled in him the attitude that it is a privilege to serve as a physician.

EXPERT CONTRIBUTORS

Iqbal "Ike" K. Ahmed, MD is currently the Medical Director of Prism Eye Institute in Mississauga and Brampton, Ontario, Canada. He is also the Head of the Ophthalmology Division at Trillium Health Partners in Mississauga, Ontario, Canada and an Assistant Clinical Professor at the University of Toronto, Ontario.

Graham D. Barrett, MBBCh, FRANZO, FRACS is a Clinical Professor at the Lions Eye Institute at the University of Western Australia. He is also the Founding and Current President of AUSCRS, Past President of APACRS, and Past President of IIIC.

David F. Chang, MD is a past president of ASCRS and current co-chair of the ASCRS Foundation. He is a clinical professor at the University of California, San Francisco, and in private practice in Los Altos, California.

Robert J. Cionni, MD is currently the Medical Director at The Eye Institute of Utah in Salt Lake City, Utah. Prior to joining The Eye Institute of Utah, he practiced for 20 years at Cincinnati Eye Institute and he recently served as President for ASCRS.

Warren E. Hill, MD, FACS has been in private practice for the past 33 years and is an Adjunct Professor of Ophthalmology and Visual Sciences at Case Western Reserve University. He has more than 140 publications, delivered 29 eponymous lectureships, and presented 805 clinical papers at both national and international meetings in 46 countries.

Anup Khatana, MD is the director of the glaucoma service at Cincinnati Eye Institute, and Volunteer Clinical Assistant Professor of Ophthalmology at the University of Cincinnati College of Medicine.

Douglas D. Koch, MD is a Professor and Allen, Mosbacher, and Law Chair in Ophthalmology at the Cullen Eye Institute of Baylor College of Medicine in Houston. He is Editor Emeritus of the *Journal of Cataract & Refractive Surgery* and Past President of the American Ophthalmological Society, ASCRS, and IIIC.

Richard L. Lindstrom, MD is the Founder and Attending Surgeon at Minnesota Eye Consultants, Clinical Professor Emeritus of Ophthalmology at the University of Minnesota, Visiting Professor at the UC Irvine Gavin Herbert Eye Institute, and Global Chief Medical Editor of *Ocular Surgery News*.

Richard J. Mackool, MD is the founder and Director of The Mackool Eye Institute and Laser Center in Queens, New York.

Samuel Masket, MD is a Past President of ASCRS, Past Member of the AAO Board of Trustees, Associate Examiner for the American Board of Ophthalmology, and Founding Partner of Advanced Vision Care in Los Angeles. He is currently the Director of Research and Fellowship Program at Advanced Vision Care.

James M. Osher, MD is a Vitreoretinal Surgeon with Cincinnati Eye Institute. He is the Assistant Clinical Professor of Ophthalmology at the University of Cincinnati and serves as Associate Director of the Vitreoretinal Fellowship.

Christopher D. Riemann, MD is a Volunteer Professor at the University of Cincinnati and Director of the Vitreoretinal Fellowship at Cincinnati Eye Institute and University of Cincinnati.

Michael E. Snyder, MD is an Associate Professor of Ophthalmology at the University of Cincinnati. He is the Chair of the Clinical Research Committee at Cincinnati Eye Institute, where he is also in private practice.

PREFACE

Two years ago, as a corneal fellow, I attended Dr. Osher's annual conference on the subject of cataract surgery—an event that he charmingly calls "Cataract Surgery: Telling it Like it Is." The name encapsulates the concept well; it is a week of intensely practical and immediately useful operative insights delivered by an all-star lineup of undisputed cataract surgery "greats." One of the sessions that week was entitled "What I Say" and featured a panel discussion of how to talk to patients in various potentially tricky situations.

After the conference, Bob was kind enough to invite me to Cincinnati where I spent 2 days listening to him talk with his patients. To date, I have never met another physician so careful and thoughtful with his words, which he employs to achieve the utmost in clarity, intelligence, and empathy. This book represents my attempt to share some of these words; that is, the metaphors and analogies (and jokes) that he regularly leverages to such great effect.

In writing this book, it quickly became apparent how much value could be added by giving voice to other esteemed surgeons and, as a result, a number of these included chapters have been "guest authored" by world experts in their special areas of accomplishment.

Transcribing these lines was a deeply rewarding experience for me; it has solidified in me a belief that we surgeons cannot reasonably harbor submillimetric concerns over the actions of our hands, and—at the same time—a casual indifference to the motions of our mouths.

—*Jack S. Parker, MD, PhD*

After 4 decades in ophthalmology, I have observed so many changes. Cataract surgery has evolved from intracapsular extraction to extracapsular to phaco with high quality IOLs that can be inserted through tiny incisions. But one thing remains constant... the requirement for effective communication. Practice patterns have also changed, and physicians are under greater pressure to see more patients in less time. Selecting the best words in combination with sincerity and unspoken body language is more important than ever as we try to explain, manage, and reassure patient after patient. Like Dr. Dick Lindstrom, I had the opportunity to spend a year with a communication master, Dr. J. Lawton Smith, the renowned neuro-ophthalmologist from Bascom Palmer. He had a magical way with words, establishing himself as a legendary teacher. I can still hear him preaching "we cannot always cure; but with our words, we can always comfort."

Throughout my career I have always enjoyed talking with my patients. Another giant ophthalmology mentor, my father Dr. Morris Osher, taught me to treat every patient with kindness and respect as if they were close family. Forty years later, I have not had a single lawsuit, and still love most every patient encounter. I hope some of these patient dialogues will prove worthwhile and help you in your everyday communication.

—*Robert H. Osher, MD*

FOREWORD

Communication skills are critically important to every physician. Good communication skills are part of the so called "art" of medicine, but they are an "art" that can be learned. A greatly skilled physician with very poor communication skills and a poor bedside manner will frequently struggle with situations that a less skilled surgeon with excellent communication skills manages with ease. When I was a fourth-year medical student, I was blessed to spend 6 weeks with Malcolm McCannel, MD. Dr McCannel is an ophthalmologist from a former generation that considers good communication with patients and colleagues a top priority. This time watching a master communicate with his patients was very impactful on my career.

The consequences of poor communication can be devastating, as evidenced in the famous 1967 movie *Cool Hand Luke,* which won (the then very young) Paul Newman an Oscar. As the prison riot escalated in the movie and many guards and prisoners were hurt or killed, the crusty warden concluded: "What we have here is failure to communicate!" Many studies, including those by the American Academy of Ophthalmology's Ophthalmic Mutual Insurance Company (OMIC) and my insurance carrier Minnesota Medical Insurance Company (MMIC), have proven that good communication is the most effective deterrent against malpractice lawsuits.

Good communication skills are verbal and nonverbal and include the environment where the communication occurs. The good communicator is also a careful and perceptive listener. Nonverbal body language, eye contact, hand gestures, and nonthreatening touching are important. The best verbal communication is clear, concise, friendly, and presented with confidence. Empathy, respect, and open mindedness with awareness of cultural differences is important. Still, for every culture it is a truism that patients do not care how much you know until they know how much you care.

We are fortunate that one of today's greatest communicators and teachers Robert H. Osher, MD and his protégé Jack S. Parker, MD, PhD (along with a group of extraordinarily talented and experienced colleagues) have created for us a book on effective patient communication for ophthalmology's most common procedure, cataract surgery. This book, published by SLACK Incorporated, will enhance the skills of every ophthalmologist as they deal with routine and complicated cataract surgery, as well as patients ranging from nice to nasty. This is a book worth owning, and to gain its full value it needs to be read and referenced more than once.

—*Richard L. Lindstrom, MD*

INTRODUCTION

Want to improve your cataract surgery results without investing a penny in expensive new technology or traveling the globe to hear the latest surgical breakthrough? Consider upgrading a piece of equipment you already possess—an indispensable organ that can make your life either miserable or more enjoyable... your mouth. The truth is, the words you say—before, after, and even during the operation—influence patient satisfaction in a big way, probably as much as the objective quality of your work.

Knowing *exactly* the right thing to say is a superpower, or at least a *force-multiplier*. Patients flock to doctors who are skillful communicators, and that depends critically on whether you've considered what you're going to say in difficult situations ahead of time, not when you're on the spot. Knowing in advance which words to use is analogous to knowing how to manage a complication before it occurs... the results are inevitably better.

In these pages, we provide our conversational scripts for use in such situations. Overwhelmingly these are the words of Dr. Osher, updated and honed over a 40-year career in ophthalmology. It is a rare occasion when Dr. Osher fails to receive an "excellent" on the quality care surveys at CEI (Cincinnati Eye Institute). We don't claim they're the only, or even the best things to say, merely that these carefully selected words have helped Dr. Osher to connect, to motivate, to manage expectations, and to build strong and trusting patient relationships.

Alongside our own remarks, we've also included bonus commentary from an all-star lineup of expert ophthalmic surgeons and famously effective communicators who likewise weigh-in with "what they say" to their own patients. We hope you enjoy.

—*Jack S. Parker, MD, PhD*

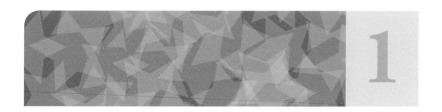

PREOPERATIVE
CONVERSATIONS

Osher RH, Parker JS.
What I Say: Conversations That Improve the
Physician–Patient Relationship (pp 1–48).
© 2019 Taylor & Francis Group.

THE HIGH MYOPE

Robert H. Osher, MD

As I'm reviewing the diagnostic measurements, before I start the exam, I look at the patient and ask if they are aware that they have a long eye. Invariably, they respond that no one has ever told them that. As a courtesy to their previous doctors, I reply:

> That's because the testing we do for cataract surgery is the only way to know this.

Then I look at the patient, point to my eye, and say the following.

> I have a normal-sized eye, about the size of a golf ball. Your eye is more like a watermelon. Because it's so large from front to back, the retina—the most important part of the eye, the film of the camera—is stretched, like a lady's belly at 9 months of pregnancy. So, you are more likely to develop a retinal tear or retinal detachment, *unrelated to surgery,* at any point in your life.

Now I would point to myself.

> For me, I would have to get hit in the eye to develop a retinal tear or detachment, but you might be walking down the street whistling Dixie and it could happen. So, I like to take a moment with all of my long-eye patients, which by the way is the reason you are nearsighted, to review the 3 important warning symptoms.

At this point, I put up my 3 fingers, point to the first finger.

> Flashes off to the side like it's the 4th of July, but it's not. This is the first warning symptom.

Pointing to the second finger, I say,

> A sudden shower of floaters (not an occasional floater, which is normal) but an epidemic of gnats is the second warning sign.

Pointing to the third finger, I say,

> The final warning sign is a curtain that covers any part of your vision. If you develop flashes, floaters, or a curtain, you have to call our office and say that Dr. Osher explained that I have

a long eye, I have a warning symptom, and I need to be seen today!

At this point I gently slap the back of one hand into the palm of the other to emphasize the point.

Next, I check in my chart that I have explained to every axial myope the increased risk of retinal tear/detachment, and I have given the highly myopic patient the appropriate informed consent.

After the exam, I will tackle the confusing topic of refractive targeting. If the patient has a unilateral cataract with more than 2.5 D (diopters) of myopia in the fellow eye and uses spectacles rather than contact lenses, the conversation transitions to postoperative refractive goals.

> Human beings need 2 eyes working together in order to enjoy depth perception, the same way we need 2 ears working together to enjoy stereo sound. But if the 2 eyes are very different, they will not work together. If you are wearing a thick glass to correct your nearsightedness in the unoperated eye, I cannot select an intraocular lens (or IOL) that will entirely eliminate your nearsightedness, or the difference will be confusing to your brain. This would be like holding up an ice cube in front of just one eye—I could not fuse the images together. So, we will need to leave a little nearsightedness following surgery, if you intend to continue using your glasses.

> You may want to consider trying a contact lens or even consider a refractive surgery like LASIK or clear lens surgery for the unoperated eye, if you would like the idea of being less dependent upon glasses. If we reduce the nearsightedness in the unoperated eye, we could try our best to select an intraocular lens that would eliminate almost all of your nearsightedness and leave you with better vision in the operated eye, even when you are not wearing glasses following surgery. However, if you do not mind wearing your glasses, we can reduce your nearsightedness to a fraction of what it is now, and you would not have to fiddle with a contact lens or consider surgery on the eye without a cataract.

If the patient has bilateral cataracts with more than 3 D of myopia and uses spectacles, then the first portion of the myopia conversation on Page 2 still applies. However, I go on to say:

The downside of having a long eyeball is that you have a very small risk of developing a retinal tear or detachment at some point in your life. However, the upside is that we can correct the majority of your myopia by selecting an intraocular lens that will put most of your prescription inside the eye. But if you choose to see more clearly at distance, which is what most patients choose, there will be too much of a difference in the thickness between your right and left lenses in your glasses following surgery. Imagine window glass on the side that we operate and your same thick lens in front of your unoperated eye—your brain will not be able to fuse the images. Therefore, in the interval before surgery in your first eye and operating upon the second eye, you will have a condition called Aniseikonia that prevents you from being able to use both eyes together. I want to emphasize that you cannot simply pop out the one lens in your glasses on the side that had surgery! You will need to either use just one eye at a time until we operate on the second eye or try to wear a contact lens in the eye that still has the cataract. Most patients will easily adapt to using only one eye during this interval and I expect the operated eye to be your preferred eye after just several days of healing. If you need to see up close, you can use the unoperated myopic eye or you can get a temporary reading glass for your new eye. When the second cataract is removed, both eyes will automatically work together. I know this is a very confusing discussion, but you are going to be very happy with the way that you are seeing the world after surgery.

At this point, I check a box that says I explained Aniseikonia which is next to the box that indicates that I have explained the increased risk of retinal tear/detachment.

SIGNIFICANT ASTIGMATISM

Robert H. Osher, MD

Before I walk into the exam room, I lift the chart out of the rack and quickly peruse the diagnostic measurements. Because I'm in an academic practice, on one sheet I can see the manual Ks, the IOL master Ks, the Lenstar Ks, the iTrace Ks, the Pentacam Ks, and the Atlas topography. In a moment, I know whether or not the patient is a toric lens candidate. After walking into the room, introducing myself to the patient and, while shaking their hand, I ask if they are aware that they have significant astigmatism. This question is analogous to a magician forcing a card on an unknowing bystander because he already has the answer. Regardless of what the patient says, I quickly start my brief explanation as follows:

> Your cornea is supposed to be round like a marble. But yours is warped like a spoon. You didn't get the basketball-shaped cornea when you were born; you got the football-shaped cornea, and this is called astigmatism. I can show it to you.

At this point I hold up their topography (Figure 1-1).

> This represents your cornea. Here's where your nose is and here's your eyebrow. Think of a bird flying over an island. When a bird flies over this island *[pointing]*, it's ok to see the blue ocean around it, and if there's no astigmatism the island is green and plush. Your island—your cornea—has these high red mountains.

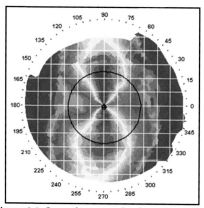

Figure 1-1. Corneal topography shown to patient.

I point to the steepening.

    That's what your astigmatism looks like.

At that point, I usually don't need to provide more explanation about astigmatism, although I will explain the option of a toric IOL in the discussion after the examination. Most patients do not want to have mountains on their cornea, and an astigmatism-correcting lens is what they will probably choose if either they do not like wearing glasses or if they can afford the investment.

If the patient asks if this means he or she won't have to wear glasses, I reply:

> No, it means that I'm going to try my best to reduce your astigmatism, which will give you clearer vision when you're not wearing your glasses. **But** we never promise that you'll never wear glasses, for 2 reasons. First, we only make lenses in steps: like 21, 22, 23… You might be a 21.36 and we don't make that lens. So, we have to err up or down, leaving you with a little nearsightedness, farsightedness, or astigmatism. Second, every patient heals differently, so you may have to wear glasses some of the time. But, you should notice a huge improvement in your vision following surgery.

THE PATIENT ON FLOMAX OR SIMILAR TYPE OF INTRAOPERATIVE FLOPPY IRIS SYNDROME-PRODUCING DRUG

Robert H. Osher, MD

Another epidemic. Some days it seems that every patient has taken Flomax, even the women. I believe this represents a philosophical conflict: to see or to pee!

> I noticed that you have taken Flomax, and I want to tell you bluntly that this drug can be lethal to the iris. As you know, the iris is the colored part of your eye that surrounds the pupil, much like the donut surrounds the hole in the center. But instead of having the consistency of a donut, patients who have taken Flomax have an iris that is floppy and behaves more like a parachute. Not only does the pupil fail to open very well during surgery, it actually gets smaller. Taking out the cataract can be as challenging as taking out an elephant through a mouse hole! We use some medications which can help, but occasionally we will need to put in a small thread-like device which helps to open the pupil enough to safely remove the cataract (Figure 1-2). You don't need to stop your Flomax if your urologist or internist believe that this medicine is helping you because it has already affected the iris and its effect cannot be reversed. We encounter a floppy iris frequently because so many patients use Flomax, and we've gotten very experienced at removing the cataract safely.

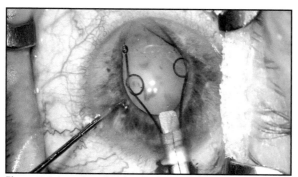

Figure 1-2. Insertion of Malyugin ring on Osher injector.

THE PATIENT ON ANTICOAGULATION

Robert H. Osher, MD

It is our policy to avoid retrobulbar anesthesia if the patient is using anticoagulant medications. The anesthesia team may favor topical anesthesia, but I may decide to use a peri-bulbar anesthetic if the patient has had pre-existing photophobia, anxiety, or may be less likely to cooperate.

I want to spend just a moment talking about your use of blood thinners. I am not qualified to decide whether or not you should continue or stop your medication, but you should discuss this with your internist. Naturally, there is a slight increase in the risk of bleeding when a patient is on blood-thinning drugs, but we are usually pretty good about avoiding blood vessels when we make our tiny 2-mm incision. On the day of surgery, you will talk to the anesthesia team about how they will numb the eye, which may or may not leave you with a little bruising. Other than that, I expect your operation to be routine and successful.

PSEUDOEXFOLIATION SYNDROME

Robert H. Osher, MD

I will usually take a picture of the white, flaky material during the exam and point this out to the patient during our discussion. Then I will say:

> This whitish stuff is like a fine powder, almost like dandruff, and we see this commonly in patients with a cataract. This stuff has a long name, pseudoexfoliation, and in some patients it can make things more difficult during—and even after—surgery.
>
> The powder is sticky, and it may prevent the pupil from dilating well, which can make removing the cataract more challenging, like taking apart an elephant through a mouse hole. It actually represents degeneration of some structures that we call zonules, which are the trampoline strings that hold the cataract inside the eye. If these trampoline strings are too weak, the lens may become unstable during surgery, or the artificial lens that we implant could become loose or dislocate even years after surgery. Fortunately, we are pretty good at fixing these problems, but it does raise your risk slightly for complications.
>
> The other thing that this powder can do is clog up the drainpipes of the eye, and that can be associated with glaucoma. You'll need to be pretty religious about routine, periodic exams in the future, just to keep an eye on your pressures. I have to tell you these things for good informed consent, but I operate on lots of patients like you with excellent results, and I will always tell you exactly where we stand.

POSTERIOR POLAR CATARACT
Robert H. Osher, MD

Prior to the article written by Douglas Koch, MD and myself in 1990 (Osher RH, Bernard C-Y, Koch DD. Posterior polar cataracts: A predisposition to intraoperative posterior capsular rupture. *J Cataract Refract Surg.* 1990;16:157-162), these cataracts (Figure 1-3) were not operated on, but rather followed by conservative observation. Even though we experienced a higher risk of an open capsule, the benefit of surgery clearly outweighed the risk in patients whose axial opacity was consistent with their compromised vision. While these patients often saw well with a dilated pupil in a darkened examining room, they were usually legally blind on a bright day or when encountering oncoming headlights at night.

> You have a very unusual type of cataract, which we call posterior polar. You've actually had this cataract since birth, although it may have gotten worse as an adult. It looks like a snowball; and although it's not a big cataract, it's right smack in the middle of the lens as if someone threw a snowball right in the middle of your windshield. The reason this is a challenging type of cataract is that the lens of the eye is surrounded by a very thin membrane like plastic wrap that we call the capsule. This is what holds the lens intact—like the skin of the grape which encloses the pulp. This membrane is usually about 4 microns thick and surprisingly strong.
>
> However, the posterior polar cataract has the thinnest possible membrane, only 1 micron, and sometimes even no microns thick, so these can be a real challenge. Rarely, the cataract will fall through the defective membrane and drop to the back of the eye. In that case, an additional procedure by a retinal specialist could be necessary. But even with the increased risk of complications, most patients do fine and you'll know exactly where we stand. I'm very optimistic and I'll do my best for you.

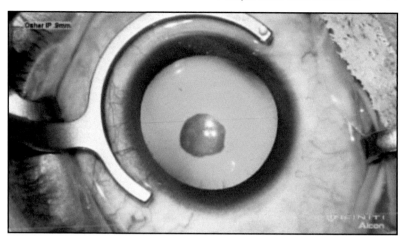

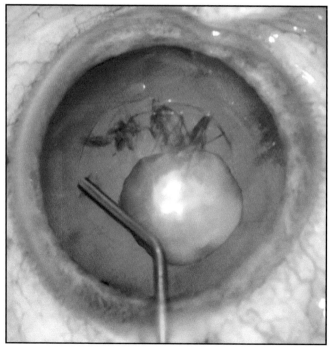

Figure 1-3. Posterior polar cataracts.

HISTORY OF PREVIOUS TRAUMA

Robert H. Osher, MD

Trauma covers such a wide injury spectrum, from minimal damage to total destruction of an eye. In my practice, I see the less severe cases with a remote history, while the vitreoretinal team tackles the more acute open globes.

I have to give you a guarded prognosis because of the previous trauma. An injury to the eye is a little like an iceberg: we can only see the tip and we never know what we are going to encounter during surgery. Sometimes we find damage to the lens of the eye that has become the cataract and it is unstable, loose, or even ruptured. Sometimes we find that the spider web-like structures called the zonules which hold the lens in place are damaged and the cataract can actually fall into the back of the eye and require an additional operation. Sometimes we find that the retina is damaged, and the eye is not capable of recovering 20/20 vision after surgery. It is also possible that a patient who has had a significant injury can develop either glaucoma or retinal swelling, a tear, or a detachment years after an injury. So, to be perfectly honest, an eye that has a previous history of trauma has a greater risk of complications during, soon after, or even years after cataract surgery. The good news is that most patients after an injury have successful cataract surgery and the odds are strongly in your favor.

HISTORY OF PREVIOUS VITRECTOMY
Robert H. Osher, MD

With 10 vitreoretinal surgeons in our practice, I see these patients frequently. Lens-iris diaphragm retropulsion syndrome (LIDRS) is to be expected in surgery, and it is easily managed by gently depressing the anterior capsule to allow infusion fluid to gain access to the retroiridal space, breaking the reverse pupillary block.

I want to emphasize that you no longer have a *virgin* eye because it has already been operated on, so I need to explain the increased risks after a previous vitrectomy.

First, the vitreous jelly, which is gone, served to support the retina—the most important part of the eye. Now that that support is gone, it is more likely that you can develop a retinal tear, detachment, hemorrhage, or even swelling of the retina at any point in your life, regardless of whether or not you have cataract surgery. We'll review the warning symptoms with you.

(See *The High Myope* section at the beginning of this chapter.)

When your vitrectomy was being performed, the retina surgeon had to pass the instruments very close to the lens of the eye, and it is always possible that the instrument may have nicked the lens and damaged it. If we find that a hole has been accidentally made in the lens, or through the spider-web like structures that hold the lens, then the cataract surgery can be more difficult, and I have to manage this more challenging situation. Rarely, I may even need to ask the retina surgeons for help.

If we do encounter damage to the cataract or the structures that support it, we may need to implant a different type of artificial lens than the one we intended for you.

Finally, the absence of the vitreous jelly also makes the selection of the intraocular lens less accurate, so you should plan on wearing a thin pair of glasses after surgery. The good news is that the vast majority of patients who have undergone previous vitrectomy enjoy a very successful result following cataract surgery, and I will do my best for you.

HISTORY OF PREVIOUS
LASIK, PRK, OR RK

Robert H. Osher, MD

It's like an epidemic…

I want to say a few words about your previous LASIK (or PRK/ RK). The good news is that this operation was able to reduce your nearsightedness. The not-so-good news is that previous corneal surgery makes it impossible to be as accurate in selecting the intraocular lens.

You see, we pick out the intraocular lens based on 2 things: the length of the eye (which we can measure in 100ths of a millimeter), and the curve of the cornea. After you have had corneal surgery, instead of having a nice, smooth curve like a marble, yours is more like a golf course with hills and valleys.

At that point, I show them the topography and point out the colors and the scale which goes from blue to red.

Therefore, I tell every single patient like you who has had LASIK, PRK, or RK that we can remove the cataract safely, but the selection of the replacement lens is going to be a *guestimation*. Consequently, you should just plan on wearing glasses following surgery. By removing the cataract, you will see very well, and although we will do our best to guess the correct power of the implant, you will see your best when you are wearing your glasses.

THE PATIENT INTERESTED IN PRESBYOPIC CORRECTION

Michael E. Snyder, MD

Author's note from Robert H. Osher, MD: Mike Snyder, MD joined Bob Cionni, MD and myself on the cataract team at CEI. For years, we shared the most challenging patients referred with traumatic cataracts, loose zonules, aniridia, posterior polar cataracts, and dislocated IOLs. Mike not only has an amazing surgical repertoire, but he also has a gift of communication with these difficult patients who need a clear understanding of their risks, benefits, and surgical options.

The number one complication of cataract surgery is presbyopia. Let that settle in for a moment.

When one begins with this in mind, a better understanding of the patient informs the conversation. As a lifetime emmetrope, presbyopia was an unhappy awakening for me. But that's just me; many of you may feel differently. My bespectacled myopic peers often don't viscerally appreciate my perturbation with my readers.

Discussions of IOL aim and presbyopia often are (and should be) more of a dialogue than a soliloquy. The conversation is different for a myope than an emmetrope or a hyperope. It is a very different discussion for the pre-presbyope that has not yet experienced the inconvenience of lacking accommodation. Nonetheless, I will try to outline to you how I approach the discussion of presbyopia in the about-to-be-pseudophakes in my practice.

I will presume for the sake of this section that the individual has a cornea from which we expect a spherical outcome or that toricity has been discussed as a separate point already and that the patient wishes to have any existing astigmatism corrected, since I believe that there is already a chapter on this topic.

I like to describe to patients that there are 3 functional ranges of focus: distance, intermediate, and near.

Distance is typically considered to be things like street signs and the TV on the other side of the room. Intermediate range is more like the dashboard, dinner plate, kitchen sink, or countertop. And near is typically a book, magazine, or cell phone. A single-focus implant lens will usually provide good vision at one of these ranges, and one would expect to need corrective lenses (glasses) for the other 2 ranges in any given eye.

Some people might choose one eye at one range and the other eye at another range. This has the advantage of covering 2 of the 3 ranges, but there will still be one point of focus that will likely still need help. This is called monovision. Some people love it, others may hate it. The advantage of monovision is a broader range providing 2 of the 3 focal zones without glasses, the disadvantage is that the 2 eyes do not work together. You know you better than I know you; you can think about whether you would like this or not.

Then I look at their face and try to gauge their emotional feedback. Then I describe:

There are some implants that are designed for a broader range of focus with the 2 eyes working together. Multifocal implants have concentric zones that are designed to achieve this.

This is the point at which I show them an oversized model of a multifocal IOL and circle my finger along the echelettes.

The advantage of these lenses is that they provide a broader range of vision to the majority of patients. A large majority of people, once both eyes are settled, end up free of glasses for everything—but not everyone. Some folks need glasses for some tasks, it may only be for reading the finest of print in the dimmest of light; for others they may need glasses regularly. There is no perfect lens.

Because of the concentric zone design, some people may notice bothersome halos or glare, as you might imagine. Most people do not notice this, but some do. Many adapt over time, but not all; and some find it annoying. Some people decide that they do not like this kind of lens, either because of halos or glare, or because they do not like the crispness of vision, or other reasons. About 1% choose to have the implant removed and replaced. Fortunately, there is an escape hatch through which it can be done safely, although it is a trip back to the operating room if you are in that 1%.

Do remember that some IOL exchanges are also performed for negative and positive dysphotopsias in monofocal implants of every type as well.

> There are some other lenses also designed for broader range. They work, ostensibly, by flexing within the eye. These lenses provide pretty good vision for distance and about 9 out of 10 get very good intermediate vision. Roughly half are free of glasses at near, about a coin toss. In less than 1% of these implants, it can flex in a funny way.

This is where I will demonstrate a Z-syndrome in an oversized model.

> If this happens, it can distort the vision and sometimes the implant needs to be replaced. Remember how we talked about that there are no perfect implants?

> The special implants that correct for a broader range do come with an extra cost. Some of that cost is related to the intraocular lens itself, and some is related to the extra things that I will do for you with this implant—including my commitment to making you as happy as we can if we run into any challenges. God forbid, if you were to fall into the 1% and you choose to have the implant replaced, I will absorb any extra cost for you. Of course, I can make you that promise very safely, knowing that it is very unlikely that you will take me up on it!

> Certainly, if it is not a good financial choice for you, then don't pick this. Fiscal responsibility is only a bad word in Washington! Whatever you pick, I am going to do a great job for you!

Frequently, some patients will report that a friend or neighbor had a standard lens and still is free of glasses. I will tell these patients that neither of us may be fully aware of the details of that person's care, and a little less than 10% of people with a standard lens aiming for distance in each eye will end up without glasses anyhow.

> Perhaps that might be you, but the statistics are unlikely.

Now I must backtrack a bit. I feel compelled to remind the reader that not all patients are candidates for a multifocal or an "accommodating" IOL. If I have identified on exam a reason that they may not be eligible for one or both styles of IOL before the discussion, I will always inform them that there are implants that are designed for a broader range of vision.

> You may have heard about multifocal intraocular lenses. Because of your *[cornea disease, macular degeneration, advanced glaucoma, etc]*, this is not a great choice for you since the multifocal implants do not behave as well in this setting, but I wanted you to know that I am aware of them. I am just not advising this choice for you.

Similarly, I may tell a patient with a zonulopathy-like pseudoexfoliation syndrome that an accommodating implant is not a viable choice, given their underlying eye disease. It is important that patients who are not candidates for a special IOL know that these implants exist. This way they do not feel that they have been given short shrift when they hear of their friend who no longer needs glasses at all, yet they weren't offered this option. I have seen such patients in consultation for a second opinion and they are sometimes unnecessarily angry with their implanting surgeon.

As long as we remember that it is always the patient's choice as to what is likely to make them the happiest and we extract any personal judgment from the conversation, we and the patient are aligned for success, irrespective of what style of IOL is selected. Please leave thoughts of "conversion rates" outside of the exam room door. The definition of a professional is one who puts the interests of those served above his or her own personal interests.

THE PATIENT INTERESTED IN MONOVISION

Graham D. Barrett, MBBCh, FRANZO, FRACS

Author's note from Robert H. Osher, MD: Graham Barrett, MBBCh, FRANZO, FRACS is a one-of-a-kind, bona fide Renaissance man. Although he practices far away from the "civilized world" in Perth, Australia, Graham's communication skills are largely responsible for his becoming a household name in ophthalmology on 6 continents.

I am often asked for advice on how to broach the topic of monovision as a presbyopic solution. This conversation feels very natural to me, as it remains the preferred solution for my patients undergoing cataract surgery.

After explaining that cataracts (or clouding of the natural lens) is the reason for their visual difficulties, I offer surgical removal and replacement of the cloudy lens as the definitive way to resolve this issue and discuss the risks of the procedure. I ask the patient who they think determines when surgery is required and, if necessary, prompt them that it is their decision. The cataract is not "a fruit which has to ripen," and they are best able to determine whether the degree of functional impairment warrants surgical intervention.

If they want to proceed, I then discuss the type of lenses available, starting with a monofocal IOL that provides the best quality of vision but has a single focus. If distance is targeted, then they will not require glasses for distance but will require readers. I always add that despite the multiple measurements, occasionally the target refraction may not be achieved and spectacles may rarely be required for distance as well as near. I then discuss the option of multifocal IOLs with multiple or extended foci that can provide reading vision without spectacles. The compromise with this type of lens is that unwanted images such as halos or reduced contrast/quality may occasionally be troublesome for some patients. At this stage patients often ask for my advice and I explain that my personal preference is for a monofocal lens, as there is an option to target a modest level of short-sightedness in the second eye if the target for distance is achieved in the first eye. Typically, I perform surgery in the eye with the denser cataract and worse vision first. I will aim for distance regardless of dominance, as my target for near vision is modest monovision at approximately -1.25 D which maintains binocularity and steroacuity. Occasionally, if a patient is myopic or accustomed to monovision, I will target a little more myopia in the second eye of approximately -1.5 D. In addition, if I encounter a patient with the denser cataract and poorer vision in the more myopic eye in the context of longstanding high myopia and anisometropia, I will do this eye first and target myopia of -1.5 D.

The conversation regarding monovision continues after the first eye has been done at the final 4-week postoperative visit. At that stage, the operated eye typically has excellent unaided vision that I demonstrate to the patient on a Snellen chart by covering the unoperated eye using a trial frame and occluder. I then use reading material to show them that the recently operated eye is unable to read without assistance, and then insert a +1.25 lens in the trial frame of the recently operated eye. This will demonstrate that the unaided distance vision in the more myopic second eye will be impaired but the unaided near vision will be improved. I emphasize that they will still require reading correction for small print (although many will be totally independent of spectacles), but their intermediate vision for phones and computers will be excellent. I often describe the type of vision as "blended" rather than "monovision" and distinguish between "total" and "relative" spectacle freedom, as it is the latter we are trying to achieve. Patients are reassured that the vison in both eyes will be identical if and when they choose to wear spectacles. If a patient appears to lack comprehension on what is being discussed, then I would not consider them as a candidate for modest monovision. The majority of patients at this stage elect to proceed with modest monovision and have a clear understanding of what they can expect; and once again I emphasize the importance of achieving the target refraction particularly in postrefractive patients. Regardless of the outcome of the second eye, I recommend that the patients do obtain reading glasses at their last postoperative visit but only wear them if they feel necessary. Rarely a patient may occasionally require distance glasses for special circumstances, such as driving at night.

Astigmatism can impair a patient's vision, and the best outcomes and patient satisfaction with modest monovision is achieved if a patient ends up with less than 0.5 D residual astigmatism in both eyes. In order to achieve this, aim the targeted residual astigmatism to be close to zero—similar to the spherical equivalent target for distance. There is no evidence to support the suggestion that residual myopic astigmatism helps depth of focus; any observed effect is due to residual spherical equivalent myopia. I find toric IOLs, particularly low dioptric (T2) toric IOLs, essential to achieve this target and I utilize toric IOLs in approximately 85% of my patients. We are fortunate in Australia that private insurance covers the additional cost of a toric IOL. I do not charge an additional fee when using toric IOLs or performing modest monovision, so there is no additional expense incurred for patients. I decide on the requirement for a toric IOL for each patient and do not specifically discuss this as part of my conversation on IOL selection.

Although there are several alternatives to achieving spectacle independence after cataract surgery, I have found the strategy of modest monovision with monofocal IOLs to be remarkably successful. Patients are highly satisfied with the outcomes and there is less concern with changes in refraction and declining macular function that can occur with age. The conversation as I have detailed is straightforward and the approach does not require the careful screening, patient selection, and relatively complex explanations that are often required with other types of IOLs.

I WANT MY CATARACT REMOVED BY LASER

Samuel Masket, MD

Author's note from Robert H. Osher, MD: Still, after 4 decades, we continue to learn from Samuel Masket, MD. This meticulous surgeon and consummate clinician demonstrates his exceptional communication skills in his writing, his lectures, and in his compassionate patient care.

Yes, it's true that we can use the femtosecond laser to help remove your cataract. The laser automates some of the steps of the surgery that we typically do by hand. That's what it does, and the procedure is basically the same; we still must enter the eye to remove the cloudy lens and replace it with a man-made artificial lens. The laser does not change the surgical steps, although it does them with great precision. However, in some particular cases, the laser can make the surgery somewhat safer and more reproducible. I prefer to use the laser in certain situations (very dense cataracts, shallow anterior chambers, Fuchs Dystrophy, weak zonular fibers, and special capsule conditions such as posterior polar cataract). And the laser can help correct astigmatism. In routine cataract surgery, however, I don't think that the laser has specific benefits. However, if you enjoy cutting edge technology, we will use the laser. Please note that it may carry an out of pocket expense for you that is generally not covered by insurance.

LOWERING EXPECTATIONS FOR SPECTACLE-FREE VISION

Robert H. Osher, MD

It is always better to under-promise, and then the patient is pleasantly surprised when they achieve excellent uncorrected vision.

> Mr. or Mrs. _____, although our technology and our formulas for selecting IOLs have improved greatly, we still cannot promise that you will not need to wear glasses following surgery. First of all, we make the implants in limited powers, for example: 21, 22, and 23. You might need a 21.36 to see perfect, and we don't make that lens. So, we err up or down to the closest power available. This means that there will probably be some residual nearsightedness, farsightedness, or astigmatism that will allow your vision to improve when you put on a thin pair of glasses. Moreover, everyone heals differently, and even a fraction of a millimeter in the implant position when the eye has healed can make a significant difference in the need for glasses. I am confident that your vision will improve once the cataract has been removed, but you should not expect to see crystal clear when you are not wearing glasses.

COEXISTING BLEPHARITIS

Robert H. Osher, MD

This simple regimen has been effective in improving the hygiene of the lashes and, consequently, reducing the risk for surgical infection. I will typically refer patients with significant blepharitis, Meibomian gland dysfunction, or a tear deficiency to one of our subspecialty clinics for these chronic conditions. I have only encountered infectious endophthalmitis in one patient during 40 years, and this patient was immunosuppressed with ocular cicatricial pemphigoid and developed the same complication following surgery in the first eye in Boston. My surgical routine is compulsive, covering every lash with a split drape and a rigorous prep using povidone iodide. Fluid is removed from the lacrimal lake with a cellulose sponge and any exposed skin on the lateral canthus is covered with a steri-strip. Even though the evidence may be debatable, I continue to prescribe a preoperative ointment to the lashes and a postoperative topical antibiotic.

> Mr. or Mrs. _____, when I examined your eyelids under the microscope, you have a lot of secretions and debris surrounding each eyelash. I realize you can't see this when you look into a mirror, but it is very obvious using the high magnification of the microscope. We see this condition that we call blepharitis quite commonly, but I do not like to see it in patients who are going to undergo cataract surgery because these secretions can harbor bacteria—and bacteria can cause infection. The eyelashes are the very next neighborhood to the eye and we cannot take any chances. I am going to recommend a few things that are quite easy to do. First, pick up any baby shampoo and every day when you take your shower, lather the shampoo up and clean your eyelashes like this.

I show them how to do it.

> You don't have to clean the eyeball or the eyelids, just the lashes. If you do this every day between now and surgery, you will have the cleanest lashes in town! We are also going to give you an ointment to apply to your lashes for several evenings before surgery. If this condition doesn't improve, I would be happy to refer you to our blepharitis clinic, but I'm optimistic this won't be necessary.

Coexisting Dry Eye

Robert H. Osher, MD

Given the age of our cataract population, it is not surprising that many patients have a tear deficiency. Fortunately, in my referral practice most of these patients are being managed very well without my less knowledgeable intervention. If the patient has a bone-dry eye, I will refer this patient to our dry eye clinic. However, I will often see a patient with superficial punctate keratopathy involving the lower quarter of the cornea (especially with proptosis) or a markedly rapid tear breakup time (TBUT). While I may discourage the patient from choosing a multi-focal lens, I am comfortable with the following brief discussion.

> Mr. or Mrs. _____, during my examination, I noticed that your eyes appear quite dry. We see this in many of our senior citizens; after all, our skin dries out and we get wrinkles, our joints dry out and we get arthritis, and our eyes become dry because we just don't produce the quantity or quality of tears that we made when we were younger. Without that layer we call the tear film, your eyes may feel sandy or irritated. If the tears are really scarce, even your vision can be blurred. I am going to give you several samples of artificial tears and you can use these as much as you wish with no harmful effects. Just don't use the tears at the same time as your other drops because I don't want the tears to wash away the cataract medications. This may be all that the desert needs… a little bit of moisture. But if you're no better after trying these drops, I will be happy to refer you to our dry eye clinic where we have lots of options to help you.

COEXISTING EPITHELIAL BASEMENT MEMBRANE DYSTROPHY

Robert H. Osher, MD

If the patient has severe apical involvement and there is considerable astigmatism, I will send the patient to the corneal service for a superficial keratectomy. I have actually seen 4 D of astigmatism completely disappear when keratometry was repeated after superficial keratectomy.

> Mr. or Mrs. _____, when I look at the cornea—the window of your eye—under the microscope, I see a condition that many of us call map-dot fingerprint dystrophy. This is a very common condition where the cornea, which is supposed to be smooth like a marble, actually looks like the surface of the moon. It almost looks like somebody left a fingerprint or etched a map on the surface of the cornea. These squiggly little lines usually mean nothing, but they can occasionally be associated with some mild irritation or discomfort. Rarely, it can even look like a golf course with some hills and valleys which cause significant astigmatism. I do not anticipate any problems with this condition when we perform your cataract surgery, but I wanted you to be aware of it because I like to tell my patients everything.

COEXISTING KERATOCONUS

Douglas D. Koch, MD

Author's note from Robert H. Osher, MD: I first met Doug Koch, MD in the early days of the American Society of Cataract and Refractive Surgery (ASCRS), formerly known as the American Intra-Ocular Implant Society (AIOIS), around 1980. Even back then, it was obvious that this soft-spoken, humble intellect would make a tremendous contribution to ophthalmology. As a teacher, researcher, surgeon, and as a human being, Doug has reached the pinnacle in every category.

As you know, in addition to your cataract, you have a condition called keratoconus. Keratoconus is a thinning of the cornea that causes the cornea to take on an irregular shape. This irregular shape ranges from mild (having only minimal effect on your vision) to severe (requiring special hard contact lenses or even corneal transplantation).

In a mild case I would say:

In your case, the keratoconus is fairly mild. By looking at your past records, it is apparent that your keratoconus is stable. You have also indicated that you want the best possible vision without glasses. You have astigmatism in your cornea that looks like it can be treated by inserting a toric IOL implant, which is an implant with a standard design that also provides astigmatism correction. I think that this would be a good option for you, since you have no plans to wear a contact lens and your keratoconus is stable. I do not recommend a multifocal lens implant, since this could result in poor vision in your case. I do want to point out that the calculations for your lens implant are more challenging than in eyes with normal corneas. So, even if we correct your astigmatism perfectly, you could be near- or farsighted enough that glasses might be needed to get best vision.

In a severe case I would say:

In your case your keratoconus is fairly advanced, and wearing a special contact lens is required to get the best vision. In this situation, I recommend surgery with a standard IOL implant, which will work very well with your contact lens. It will also work well should you need corneal transplantation in the future if your keratoconus gets too severe (Figure 1-4).

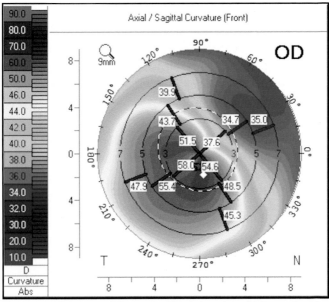

Figure 1-4. Curvature of the cornea. This is how I would discuss it with a patient: *This is an image that shows the curvature of your cornea. A normal cornea would appear mostly green with similar colors on opposite sides of the center. In your case, the region in upper right is blue, showing that your cornea there is very flat, whereas the zone down and to the left is red, indicating that your cornea is very steep there. To get good vision, it will almost certainly require you to wear a special contact lens, which will cover the irregularities and will provide much sharper focus. If the contact lens either is uncomfortable or does not give you good vision, then corneal transplantation may be required.*

COEXISTING FUCHS' CORNEAL DYSTROPHY

Robert H. Osher, MD

If the patient has stromal edema or a thick pachymetry measurement, I will probably refer this patient to the corneal service. However, the vast majority of these patients have only guttata. Even if the cell count is unmeasurable, I still feel comfortable using slow motion phaco with low parameters (Osher RH, Falzoni W, Osher JM. Our phacoemulsification technique. In: Buratto L, Werner L, Zanini M, Apple D, eds. *Phacoemulsification Principles and Techniques, Second Edition*. Thorofare, NJ: SLACK Incorporated; 2003:355-362), operating under OVD protection.

> When I was carefully examining the inside of your eye, I noticed that in addition to your cataract you also have a corneal condition that we call Fuchs' endothelial dystrophy. That's a lot of words but the problem is just the opposite, you don't have a lot of cells. Let me explain. The cornea, the window to the eye, is bathed by tears on the outside and fluid on the inside. You would think that the cornea would swell like a sponge and lose its transparency. But at birth, we are given a certain number of cells on the inner layer which act like little pumps and they spend a lifetime pumping these body fluids out of the cornea, so it can stay transparent like a picture window. For some unknown reason, some patients lose many of these cells and, in rare cases, the cornea might even swell, a condition we call corneal edema. We used to treat this condition by performing a corneal transplant and giving you a new cornea from a donor. More recently, we are able to simply give you a layer of new cells—which is a much easier and safer procedure. It's a very successful operation, but I'm glad to say that we usually don't need it because the vast majority of corneas with Fuchs dystrophy stay clear after cataract surgery. Still, I have to mention this to you in case you're one of the rare ones whose cornea decompensates after surgery. I've operated on many patients just like you whose vision has improved following surgery; maybe not to 20/20, but improved nevertheless.

We'll take a photograph which will tell us how many cells you have and we'll keep this on file in your record.

There's an old saying from medical school called Hickam's Dictum: "A man or a woman could have as many diseases as they darn well pleases." Fuchs' corneal dystrophy is usually not a problem; but if you're the unlucky one, it's nice to know that it's treatable. So, let's not worry about it.

COEXISTING MACULAR DEGENERATION

Robert H. Osher, MD

There's an old saying that I learned in medical school called Hickam's Dictum which states, "A man or a woman could have as many diseases as they darn well pleases!" You happen to have both a cataract in the front of the eye and some aging of the retina in the back of the eye. For the past 4 decades, I've done nothing but cataract surgery and I am not an expert at retinal problems. But, I can give you a good analogy: the eye is like a camera, with a lens in the front, and the film in the back. If the lens gets dirty, we can take it out and replace it, which is basically what cataract surgery accomplishes. However, if the film in the camera is not any good, the picture will not be clear even if you use the best replacement lens in the world. In other words, removing your cataract will only fix one of the problems and your vision may be much better, somewhat better, or possibly no better after cataract surgery. We should probably get an opinion from one of our retinal specialists about the back of your eye, but you have a significant cataract and are entitled to "gamble" for clearer vision—which most patients enjoy after surgery. The only promise that I can make is that I'm going to do my very best for you and I will work together with the specialists who are the experts in aging of the retina.

COEXISTING DIABETIC RETINOPATHY

James M. Osher, MD

Author's note from Robert H. Osher, MD: It is such an honor to practice with my son, Jamey Osher. His track record is impressive as an outstanding resident, winner of the Golden Apple Teaching Award during his retinal fellowship, and as a prodigious worker who has established one of the busiest referral practices at CEI. Patients love the way he instills confidence and reassurance into his conservations.

Cataract surgery provides a great opportunity to help patients improve their systemic control and proactively treat diabetic retinal disease.

> To achieve our goal of attaining the best visual outcome after cataract surgery, we need to make sure that your diabetic retinopathy is under the best control possible. First, that means working with your primary care physician to make sure your blood sugar and blood pressure are under ideal control. At the same time, if necessary, we can start to treat any retinopathy or retina swelling prior to cataract surgery. We do not need the retinopathy and swelling to be perfect, but we want it reasonably well-controlled prior to surgery. We also may want to use different types of retinal pictures to evaluate if any diabetic damage will limit your visual potential. We can continue to treat the diabetic retina disease immediately before and after cataract surgery to lower the risk of exacerbating these problems. This may include a combination of prolonged eye drops and/or shots in the eye. Finally, the presence of diabetic retinopathy and/or swelling may make some of our implant options less desirable, but we will work together with the cataract surgeon to determine your best options. We are going to take very good care of you, so don't worry!

COEXISTING EPIRETINAL MEMBRANE

James M. Osher, MD

In this case, combination surgery may be our best option.

In addition to your cataract, we have discovered that you also have an epiretinal membrane or ERM. This problem usually occurs with age, similar to your cataract. You can see that your forehead becomes more wrinkled with age; this same wrinkling can occur on the surface of your retina from the ERM. When the retina wrinkles, it can cause your vision to become blurry and distorted. The only way to treat an ERM that is affecting your vision is with surgery. Considering both eye problems, there are 2 ways we can proceed with the cataract surgery. The first way is to do the cataract surgery alone and not address the ERM. We will have to prolong your postoperative anti-inflammatory eye drops, since the presence of the ERM has an increased risk of inflammation in the central retina after cataract surgery. Once you've healed from surgery, we can further assess the visual significance of the ERM and determine if it needs to be removed with an additional surgery.

The second approach to the cataract surgery, and my preference, is to remove the ERM at the same time as the cataract surgery. With this plan, we kill 2 birds with 1 stone. We usually have to numb your eye differently and the surgery will take an extra 20 to 30 minutes. We will also have to be more patient waiting for your vision to improve, since you will be healing from both cataract and retina surgery. However, combination surgery works great and is probably the best option if we think the ERM is affecting your sight.

COEXISTING RISK FACTORS FOR POSTOPERATIVE CYSTOID MACULAR EDEMA

Robert H. Osher, MD

When the patient has been told about Cystoid Macular Edema (CME) prior to surgery, then it's a known possibility rather than an unexpected complication.

> Mr. or Mrs. _____, I want to mention that you have (epiretinal membrane, branch vein occlusion, previous uveitis, diabetic retinopathy), which can cause some swelling in the center of the retina following routine cataract surgery. This can occur even when your cataract surgery goes perfectly, and we really do not understand why. We work in the front of the eye (which is far away from the back of the eye), and you would think that if something happened in New York, it would not affect what's happening in Los Angeles. But even after a beautiful cataract operation, we can see some swelling that is usually temporary and resolves with the medications that we prescribe. Rarely, we will send a patient over to the retinal team, if this swelling persists and causes blurred vision. I don't want you to worry about this because it probably won't ever happen. But, if it did, we would take care of this retinal swelling the best we can.

COEXISTING OCULAR HYPERTENSION

Anup Khatana, MD

Author's note from Robert H. Osher, MD: Anup Khatana, MD is the head of the busy glaucoma team consisting of 9 subspecialists at CEI. He is an adept clinician, a superb surgeon, a talented teacher, and a real pro when talking to and managing his challenging patients.

You have high pressure in your eyes. This is called ocular hypertension. It increases the risk of developing the optic nerve damage that we call glaucoma, but the good news is that you do not have glaucoma yet. Only some people, not all, with high eye pressure go on to develop glaucoma. There is no good reliable way to know who will develop glaucoma, but regular monitoring should be able to catch it at a very early stage. Most eyes with ocular hypertension do not need treatment and can just be monitored. However, if the intraocular eye pressure rises to or above 28 to 30 mmHg, most physicians will treat the pressure with eye drops or laser therapy.

The pressure in the eye often rises in both normal patients and in those with ocular hypertension immediately after routine cataract surgery. The risk of such a pressure spike is greatest in the first 24 hours, but some eyes can develop temporary pressure elevation a few weeks later due to the steroid drops that we use to help the eye heal. At the same time, removing a cataract can lower the pressure in some eyes, often for several years. However, we don't have a sure-fire way to predict which eyes may get a pressure rise or fall after cataract surgery.

When we do cataract surgery on patients with high pressure, whether on pressure-lowering eye drops or not, we need to consider multiple risk factors to help determine how best to take care of that patient. There are few absolutes in this area, and different surgeons can differ on their approach. In general, if the pressure is not terribly high, we will add medicines right after surgery to try to prevent the pressure from further rising. If the pressure is at an uncomfortably high level even before surgery, we will usually try to treat the pressure and lower it to a safer level prior to performing cataract surgery. Although there are surgeries that can be performed and devices that can be implanted to lower the pressure at the time of cataract surgery, they are usually not performed if glaucoma is not present. In addition, most insurance carriers will not approve payment for such procedures in the absence of glaucoma damage. In extremely rare cases, the pressure may rise after cataract surgery to a level where it cannot be controlled even with medicines, and glaucoma surgery may become necessary.

COEXISTING GLAUCOMA

Iqbal "Ike" K. Ahmed, MD

Author's note from Robert H. Osher, MD: Ike Ahmed, MD has climbed the ladder of ophthalmic notoriety 2 rungs at a time. The Father of MIGS (microinvasive glaucoma surgery) has contributed as a master surgeon, an innovator, and a teacher in great demand—all with his eccentric flare and unique style.

Considering that 10% to 15% of patients undergoing cataract surgery have glaucoma or are taking IOP-lowering medications, the opportunity to manage both glaucoma and cataract is a one-time opportunity. Reducing the burden, inconvenience, compliance issues, side effects (including ocular surface/tear film), and costs of glaucoma drops is highly beneficial to all patients. The question in the past has generally been regarding what is the risk and impact on postoperative recovery and refractive status of the eye when combining cataract surgery with a glaucoma procedure. It is well-known that cataract surgery alone can provide approximately a 15% to 20% lowering of IOP. The ability to combine this with the new genre of MIGS procedures can further enhance both IOP-lowering and medication reduction/elimination with minimal additional risk or refractive alteration/postoperative recovery. Combining with subconjunctival filtration and/or trabeculectomy may be required for those with more advanced and uncontrolled glaucoma. The selection of the preferred option is based on a balance of risk, recovery, efficacy, and effort.

> As you are undergoing cataract surgery, we also have an opportunity to add a minor glaucoma procedure to help lower your eye pressure and reduce your glaucoma drops. Remember that fortunately cataract is a reversible cause of vision loss and has become a fantastic, predictable, and very safe procedure that can even enhance your vision and reduce your eye prescription or glasses dependence. However, your glaucoma is unfortunately a chronic irreversible cause of vision loss that is one of the leading causes of blindness.
>
> Now, I don't wish to scare you, but it behooves us to consider your glaucoma seriously and take steps to reduce this risk. As you know, we do this by lowering your eye pressure with eye

drops on the surface of your eye. The drops are safe, but do have a number of side effects and can impact the result of your cataract surgery, costs, as well as the issue of forgetting to put your drops in (which happens to the best of us). Furthermore, in many patients drops become less effective in controlling the pressure over time. In the past, traditional more invasive glaucoma surgeries, while potent, impacted postoperative recovery and vision. They also introduced significant early and long-term risks, making them less attractive to combine with cataract surgery.

For some patients who have very serious and aggressive glaucoma, we need to do this (considering glaucoma is permanently blinding disease). We now have a new class of "micro-invasive" or minor glaucoma procedures that, although not as potent as traditional procedures, can provide a greater chance of reducing or even eliminating your glaucoma drops after surgery than if we did cataract surgery alone—without most of the risks of traditional surgery or impacting your recovery very much. Combining with cataract surgery is an excellent place for these devices, as we are already planning on doing surgery. The pain during or after surgery is the same, as is the recovery in most patients compared to just doing cataract surgery alone. Fortunately, serious risks are very uncommon with MIGS devices. But the benefit of adding a MIGS procedure to your cataract surgery increases the chances of getting off of or at least on less glaucoma drops and improving the control of your disease and thus reducing the risk of long-term permanent vision loss.

The selection of which MIGS device we suggest is based on a combination of potency, risks, technique, and how much postoperative care is acceptable. It also leaves the door open to more aggressive glaucoma surgery should you need it. Of course, this is not a guarantee that you will be on no drops, but our studies show the added benefit of combining cataract surgery with MIGS. For example, some studies show the chance of being drop-free is doubled when combining cataract and MIGS versus doing cataract surgery alone. This is what I call a "step-wise" approach to glaucoma—starting with less aggressive/less risky procedures first, and moving to more aggressive procedures later as needed.

For these reasons, I think you be an excellent candidate to take the one-time opportunity to perform a very low-risk MIGS procedure when I am already in the eye removing your cataract. And of course, remember no matter what procedure is done regular monitoring, follow-up, and following instructions on your glaucoma medications is paramount to controlling this potentially serious disease. I have found that the prognosis (and improved quality of life) is excellent for the vast majority of patients with this approach.

THE PATIENT WITH A CATARACT SO ADVANCED, THE FUNDUS CANNOT BE VISUALIZED

Robert H. Osher, MD

I will still use my routine explanation and discussion, but I will always add the following.

> Mr. or Mrs. _____, your cataract is so advanced that it not only prevents you from seeing out, but it also prevents me from seeing in! Despite my best effort, I just cannot examine the retina behind the cataract. It would be like asking you to tell me what's at the bottom of the Ohio River, knowing that the muddy water would block your view. Therefore, I want to emphasize that you have a guarded prognosis because I really don't know if the retina is healthy or not. We will certainly be able to see into your eye after surgery, but the chances are very good that you will be able to see much better after this gigantic cataract is removed.

COMPLICATIONS IN THE FIRST EYE
Robert H. Osher, MD

This conversation depends upon what the complications were due to and will be answered differently if, for example, the patient has bilateral posterior polar cataracts vs an iatrogenic tear in the posterior capsule. Let's limit this conversation to the latter category where, for example, the patient had a complication that we do not anticipate being bilateral.

> I am very aware that you had a problem in your first eye, but I want to reassure you that I am taking every possible precaution to prevent this from occurring in the second eye. We learn a lot from the first eye and can use this information to your benefit. Although it is possible for lightening to strike twice, I can honestly say that there is no operation in all of medicine which is as safe as cataract surgery and I will do my best for you.

THE ONE-EYED PATIENT

Robert H. Osher, MD

I do believe in taking extra precautions when a patient only has one eye. I give several days of preoperative antibiotics as well as prophylactic IOP-lowering topical drops and even a weak-strength carbonic anhydrase inhibitor following surgery. I do not have any scientific evidence to back up this approach, but I do sleep better at night. After I complete the examination, I say the following.

> Mr. or Ms. _____, I have examined you very thoroughly and I am happy to say that I find no evidence of any serious disease. I agree with Dr. _____ that you have a cataract, like so many other people. But unlike others, you only have 1 good eye. Cataract surgery is the safest operation in medicine and is justified whenever a patient is unhappy with his or her vision and can no longer do the things he or she needs to do or wants to do. These guidelines apply whether you have 1, 2, or even 3 eyes! We should never rush into surgery, but if you've exhausted the conservative options like changing your glasses and you are still unhappy with your vision, then surgery is justified.

THE TERRIFIED PATIENT

Robert H. Osher, MD

I am quick to reach out and put my hand on the patient's hand, which communicates both my concern and confidence. Touch is also a good way of sealing the unspoken covenant that strengthens the surgeon-patient relationship.

> Mr. or Ms. _____, I know you are very worried and frightened about this operation—which is completely normal. In fact, if I was going to have eye surgery, I would probably feel the same way. But I'd figure out a way to do it on myself and I wouldn't worry as much! You shouldn't worry as much either because I've been doing just this operation for my entire career. The surgery is pretty quick, it's painless, and it's become the best operation in all of medicine. I'll treat you like my own family and we'll have a very good procedure. If you'd like, one of my nurses will hold your hand, and I'll be right next to you reassuring you every step of the way. Everybody feels a bit nervous before their first operation and then they're no longer frightened, and they can't wait to have their second operation. You're going to do really well.

THE NASTY PATIENT

Robert H. Osher, MD

It is rare when a patient behaves aggressively or rudely to the staff. However, this is the time when every physician should draw the "red line." I will immediately ask the patient to step into one of the examination rooms, and after closing the door I have the following conversation.

> Mr. or Ms. _____, my staff has told me that you are treating them with disrespect. This attitude cannot be tolerated in my practice. My staff works around the clock to help me and they share my devotion to each one of our patients. If they are upset, then I am upset. If you wish to remain a patient in this practice, I would suggest that you apologize for your rudeness and treat them as family, just like I treat my patients as family. Otherwise, I'm sure you can find another cataract surgeon elsewhere.

It is very infrequent when this happens, and most patients will immediately apologize and become among the nicest in the practice. However, I can recall a few rare cases when a patient chose to go elsewhere; he or she was not missed.

What's the Worst Thing That Can Happen to Me During Surgery?

Robert H. Osher, MD

The worse thing that can happen to you during surgery is for ME to die!

Here I take a pause for laughter!

And that wouldn't be very good for either of us. But, seriously, there are always risks with any surgery. In my 40 years, I've seen 1 case of blindness, 1 case of infection, 1 stroke, 1 heart attack, and (back in the old days when many of the cases were performed under general anesthesia) I even saw a patient who didn't wake up, like Michael Jackson. We don't use those kinds of anesthesia anymore and cataract surgery has become the very safest operation in all of medicine. Patients tell me that the exam today is more difficult than the actual surgery. The operation doesn't take very long, and I'll talk to you the entire time. You're going to do very well.

ROUTINE PATIENT DISCUSSION AT THE CONCLUSION OF THE INITIAL EXAMINATION

Robert H. Osher, MD

Mr. or Mrs. _____, the best news I can give you is that your eyes are healthy, and I don't see any evidence of serious disease *[if that it is the case].* I agree with your referring doctor that you have cataracts.

I have a video that explains what cataracts are and shows a brief surgical procedure that the patients have watched before entering the exam room.

I want to emphasize that cataract surgery has become the very best operation in all of medicine, but it is completely elective and entirely up to you. I always like to ask 3 questions.

Here I hold up 3 fingers and point to the first.

First, are you still happy with your vision?

Almost everyone says no, and I will proceed to the second finger. If they do say yes, I reassure them that I do not operate on happy patients and the cataracts can be managed by conservative observation until they are ready for surgery.

Second, which eye is worse?

It's important that the chief complaint and examination are consistent with their answer.

Well, I agree that cataract surgery is in your best interest. So, my third question is which implant do you want?

I realize that everyone has a different approach, but I like to open a box showing 3 plastic large-scale implants and I point to each as I say the following words (Figure 1-5).

You have 3 choices and only this one is covered by insurance—the other 2 you have to pay for out of your pocket because they are considered deluxe lenses. The first lens is

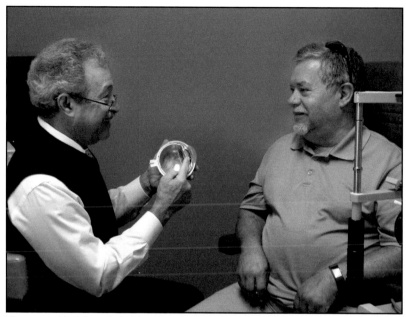

Figure 1-5. Models are helpful during patient conversations.

called a monofocal which means one focus, and you get to choose the focus. The focus can be distance *[pointing across the room]*, computer *[holding my hand at computer length]*, or reading *[moving my hand closer]*. You only can choose one, and you still may need a thin pair of glasses to correct your astigmatism.

If they choose distance, I emphasize that they will need glasses for reading and vice versa.

This lens has a great track record, a built-in sunglass, and patients are very happy.

The second choice is called T-O-R-I-C.

I spell it out for the patient.

It is exactly the same as the first lens except that it also reduces astigmatism. Patients can also choose distance, computer, or reading with this lens and it gives you the best chance of having less dependence on glasses at whatever distance you prefer.

You'll still have to wear glasses for near if you choose distance, or for distance if you choose near (just like the first monofocal), but patients love this lens. As I said, your astigmatism can be corrected by your glasses with the first lens. However, if you choose this deluxe lens, you will be responsible for $_____ out of your pocket.

The third choice is the most sophisticated of all, it is called a presbyopia-correcting lens and it allows you to see both distance and near at the same time. This is for patients who really want their best chance of not wearing glasses most of the time. For this luxury, you will responsible for $_____.

If the patient is interested in this lens, I will spend more time making sure that they understand halos, glare, and an adaption period.

Regardless of which choice you make, you are going to see better once your cataract has been removed, and I am confident that you will be very satisfied.

At this point, the patient usually has his or her mind made up and I summarize the plan verbally while I am recording it in my medical record to reflect which lens has been chosen, such as a toric lens for distance. This is the skeleton approach and does not take into consideration other discussion points like monovision, risks, and how I like to lower expectations by emphasizing that patients may still need to wear glasses because of the limited range of available implants, ie, +21, +22, +23, and you might be a +23.68, requiring a lens which we do not make. I emphasize that I have to err up or down, and because all patients heal differently a thin pair of glasses may still be necessary after surgery. I realize that many physicians have counselors who explain these things to patients, but I don't mind taking the few extra minutes to make certain that my patients are fully informed. I always end the examination by introducing the patient to my scheduling person and saying these words.

I don't want you to worry. I have been doing this a long time and I'm going to take excellent care of you. I'm a "no-hurting" doctor and the exam today is actually more difficult than the surgery.

I will often put my hand on their shoulder or reach out to shake their hand and say the following words.

It's very nice meeting you and I'll see you in surgery.

2

INTRAOPERATIVE CONVERSATIONS

Osher RH, Parker JS.
*What I Say: Conversations That Improve the
Physician-Patient Relationship (pp 49-69).*
© 2019 Taylor & Francis Group.

WHAT I SAY TO THE PATIENT BEFORE SURGERY WHEN HE OR SHE IS IN THE PREOPERATIVE AREA

Robert H. Osher, MD

Before surgery, our ambulatory surgery center (ASC) policy is that the surgeon (or the fellow) is supposed to go out to the individual pre-op bay to talk to the patient.

> Good morning, Mr. or Mrs. _____. This is Dr. Osher behind the mask! I wanted to welcome you and reassure you that I'm well prepared for your surgery today. I'm required to ask if you've had any major illness since I last saw you.

The patient shakes their head no.

> I knew that by just looking at you, but I'm required to ask that question. You're on deck, and Mary, one of our best nurses, is going to get you ready because I'm starting the patient before you and it shouldn't take too long.

Next, I look at the family member and ask the following question.

> Are you planning on watching the surgery? I'll explain to you what I'm doing, and I think you'll enjoy watching the operation.

Then, I look at the patient and usually pat their shoulder.

> I'll see you shortly and I'm going to take good care of you today.

I've televised the surgery "live" for the family to watch since 1981. I turn on the video after the incision and capsulorrhexis so the family can view and hear the explanation and reassurances that I provide from the privacy of a viewing room. Over 99% of surgeries are uncomplicated. If a complication does occur, I want the family to see how hard I work. They are typically very understanding and supportive if they've seen how I handled something unexpected. There is a red "V" on the patient's bed if I am supposed to narrate, and the families are appreciative to see the operation, which is visually riveting. Upon returning to their recovery room, family members invariably embrace the patient and say "Oh my gosh, now I understand why you couldn't see!" I like including the family in the process as it enhances the overall experience for the patient.

DRAPING AND THE CLAUSTROPHOBIC PATIENT

Robert H. Osher, MD

We've designed a drape with Beaver Visitec International (BVI) which has a translucency that extends to the other eye, so the patient can see form and motion (Figure 2-1). The drape only covers the patient from the waist up, so patients do not overheat. It is also very easy for a nurse or an anesthesia person to hold a hand. The adhesive is minimal, which contributes to patient comfort. The fluid collection bag can be torn away like a tear-away jersey at the end of the operation.

> We're going to put this little drape around the eye which will also cover any germs from your nose, mouth, and lashes, so the operation will be sterile and safe. We'll have lots of fresh air coming in under the drape and I'll put on a little music for you. The operation shouldn't take very long. I'm right here next to you, and I'll talk to you the entire time. You can tell me if anything bothers you, and I have a nurse and an anesthesia person who will be happy to hold your hand if you get nervous. You should be comfortable the entire time.

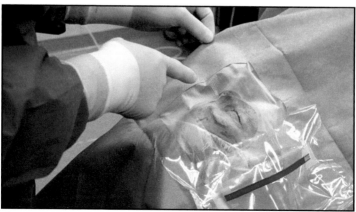

Figure 2-1. The translucent material allows the patient to see from the unoperated eye, which reduces anxiety and prevents claustrophobia.

If the patient shows signs of claustrophobic distress, I say the following.

> We're going to lift this little drape off part of your face (which we attach to an IV pole). If you open your other eye, you can see that I'm right here.

At this point, the nurse will hold the patient's hand and the anesthesia person may give something in the IV. My reassurance becomes even more frequent as I hustle to finish the surgery safely.

WHEN THE PATIENT IS ON THE OPERATING ROOM TABLE

Robert H. Osher, MD

I like to reassure the patient frequently throughout the procedure that everything is going fine. I tell them when the cataract is out, when the implant is in, when we are almost finished. Frequent communication and reassurance contribute to a positive experience for the patient.

> Hi, Mr. or Mrs. _____. It's Dr. Osher and I'm right next to you just adjusting the microscope. We're placing a few protective drapes around your eye to keep everything nice and safe and sterile. You should be completely comfortable today... tell me if there's anything that bothers you. If you feel anything unpleasant, let me know and I can give you a few more drops. If you feel like you have to move or cough, just let me know. I'm working under this high-powered microscope which is just a big magnifying glass, so a small move to you is like an earthquake to me. I've got a terrific team in this operating room and things are going to go smoothly. If it's okay with you, I'm going to be talking to your family and explaining what I'm doing. You're welcome to listen to me or to the nice, soft music in the room, but please try not to dance or sing while I'm working. We can celebrate afterwards!

THE MOVING PATIENT

Robert H. Osher, MD

If the patient is really moving, then I have planned poorly and failed to tape the patient's head which I like to do with any tremor, restless leg, or movement disorder (Figure 2-2). It is very rare when I will ask the nurses to elevate the drape and tape the head during surgery. It is even more unusual when I ask the anesthesiologist to sedate the patient, but I can recall a couple of cases where propofol was necessary to finish the case safely.

> Mr. or Mrs. _____, I know that you are doing your best to hold still while I'm operating, but I'm working under a high-power microscope and a little movement to you is like an earthquake to me. I would appreciate if you could help me by holding as still as possible. I will do my very best to finish your operation as quickly as I can, making sure that everything is perfect.

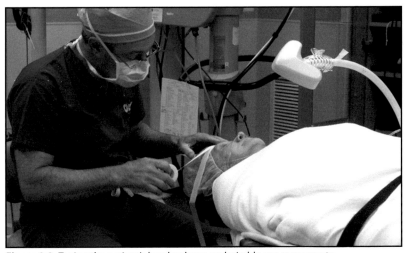

Figure 2-2. Taping the patient's head reduces undesirable eye movements.

How to Talk to the Anesthesia Person Assigned to my Room

Robert H. Osher, MD

If he or she is planning to give retrobulbar anesthesia, I always emphasize the importance of limiting the volume to no more than 3.5 cc, otherwise the anesthetic will compress the globe like 2 thumbs indenting a balloon. This is not an issue if a peribulbar block is being given. For any anesthesia (including topical), I stress the importance of minimal sedation so that the patient does not fall asleep, suddenly jerking his or her head. I want to be able to communicate with the patient the entire time, and as you know, a little too much sedation can disorient the patient with disastrous results. I like to finish our brief conversation by saying the following.

The best anesthesia in Room 5 is not general or local, it's vocal.

If there is an excessive amount of talking in the room during the procedure, I am not reluctant to say the following.

Come on gang, let's keep it down. I'm really concentrating, and everything needs to be perfect.

This is a polite way of saying, "quiet, and pay attention!" It works.

WHEN THE PHACO MACHINE FAILS... AND IT WILL, SOONER OR LATER

Robert H. Osher, MD

I always emphasize to the team that we cannot make the patient apprehensive by saying that something is not working. It is important that our conversation always reassures, rather than alarms the patient. Let's look at an example where either we lose ultrasound in the middle of the nucleus or the vacuum malfunctions.

I say the following to the staff.

> I think I'd like to change the ultrasound tip (or the tubing) because it is not testing at 100%. I want to make sure that every step in this operation is perfect, so let's take a moment and simply give me another ultrasound tip.

I say the following to the patient.

> Mr. or Mrs. _____, we are going to take just a few moments to change a piece of the equipment because I'm a perfectionist. I apologize for this little delay, but we want to make sure that every step in your operation goes exactly right.

I always apologize to the patient for the short delay and will add that everybody knows that I demand absolute perfection when I'm operating. On rare occasions we have even had to change a large piece of equipment like the whole phaco machine, which takes even longer, but patients always appreciate this brief explanation.

THE TORN POSTERIOR CAPSULE

Robert H. Osher, MD

Honesty is the best policy as long as it is accompanied by sincerity and reassurance.

> During surgery we encountered a split in the tiny cellophane-like membrane that surrounds the cataract. This membrane is only 4 microns thick (which is thinner than a red blood cell), and keeping this membrane intact is the most common challenge that we face as cataract surgeons. I was able to remove all of the cataract, and the intraocular lens is in good position, but I'm going to keep a close eye on you for the next few weeks. We may give you a few extra drops, in addition to my cell phone number. Please call me if you notice anything that does not seem right, like significant pain or any change in your vision. You will be blurry for a couple of days. This is because we don't use stitches anymore and we close these small incisions by swelling them closed.

I show my hands coming together like a clap.

> It takes a few days for the swelling to go down *[I point my thumb down]* before your vision clears up *[I turn my thumb from downward to upward]*. Judy, one of our best nurses, is going to review your instructions today, which I'll repeat tomorrow. I believe you're going to have an excellent result.

CAN'T PLACE PREMIUM INTRAOCULAR LENS

David F. Chang, MD

Author's note from Robert H. Osher, MD: David Chang, MD has been one of the brightest shining stars in cataract surgery. A gifted educator, there are few who communicate better than this talented surgeon and world-class humanitarian. His wit and humor at the podium entertain audiences around the world; and when he speaks, we all listen.

The first question is deciding when and where to fully discuss the surgical complication with the patient. Immediately following intraoperative complications, surgeons often feel emotionally shaken. This may be compounded by feeling time pressure after falling significantly behind schedule. However, trying to rush through the inevitable questions will only intensify the frustration and anxiety of patients and their families. It is best to postpone this potentially difficult and lengthy discussion until later that same day in the office. Therefore, I send the patient to the recovery area with instructions for the staff to fetch their family and to keep them at the bedside until I'm able to come out. If alternating between 2 ORs, I then operate on the patient already prepped and waiting in the next room.

In the recovery area, I first tell the patient and his or her family that the surgery was unexpectedly difficult, and that I would like to examine the eye in my office later that afternoon as a precaution and to be sure that the patient is comfortable. I reassure them that during this first check up, we will have plenty of time to discuss what happened and to review the postoperative instructions. This allows me to postpone the discussion until I have more time to spend with the patient and their family. It conveys my concern for the patient while recognizing the need to have a discussion that isn't rushed. I add that the sedation, which can cloud the patient's thinking and memory, will have worn off by that time. I schedule this office appointment at the end of the clinic day in order to allow plenty of time to answer questions in a relaxed and empathetic manner.

Besides educating the patient and answering questions, my goals are:

1. To be reassuring, patient, and empathetic

2. To provide an understandable explanation about what happened

3. To acknowledge their disappointment, anxiety, inconvenience, and fears

4. To apologize that they are having this unexpected and unpleasant experience

5. To explain what will happen next

6. To convey optimism about the prognosis

> You may recall from my literature that the cataract/human lens is surrounded by a very thin, cellophane-like membrane called the capsule. Tiny fibers hold and suspend the lens and its surrounding capsule in the eye, and we try to preserve and use the capsule along with the supporting fibers to hold the artificial lens implant in place. As a result, the artificial lens permanently occupies the same location as the original natural lens. My brochure also explained that in order to remove the cataract through the tiniest incision possible, it is broken up into a dozen or more pieces that are small enough to be gently suctioned out of the eye.

> We surgeons go into every cataract surgery knowing that on rare occasions, despite our best efforts, the capsule or its supporting fibers called "zonules" may split during the fragmenting and removal of the cataract. In your case, the back part of the capsule split, but not the front. The problem is that the multifocal lens we had planned to use will not work well unless it is perfectly centered. If it isn't, there is an increased risk of glare and blur that won't be corrected by eyeglasses. Slight amounts of tilting or imperfect centering won't be noticeable with a conventional single focus lens, however. Therefore, I

had to make a careful decision. It was very tempting to try placing the multifocal lens implant, knowing how disappointed you would probably be if I could not. However, I had to stop and ask myself what I would want if I were the patient in this situation. I decided that the risk of a poor outcome was too high with the multifocal lens, and that placing a standard single focus lens was the safest thing to do. I was able to use the part of the capsule that was not split to hold the lens implant and I'm very pleased with how secure it looks as I examine you right now.

I know that this must be surprising and disappointing for you, and I am very sorry that I wasn't able to put in the lens implant that you had preferred. However, your prognosis is still excellent, and even though you may have to wear eyeglasses more often than you had wanted, we won't have the risk of a tilted or off-center multifocal lens.

CAN'T PLACE ANY
INTRAOCULAR LENS

David F. Chang, MD

Rather than saying that the capsule tore, I say that I discovered a split in the capsule. A tear has a more negative connotation in my opinion—perhaps the result of a reckless or clumsy action. I apologize for the stress and inconvenience that they are experiencing, but I don't apologize for my actions, which could imply an admission that I made a bad mistake or did something very wrong. I try to avoid assigning blame, eg, you suddenly moved at the wrong time, the anesthesiologist over-sedated you, the equipment wasn't working properly, the nurse loaded the injector incorrectly, or the lens must have had something wrong with it. *Assigning blame elsewhere may defend my competence, but still implies that the complication was preventable. This makes it harder for the patient to accept what has happened.* Finally, I mention that I specifically thought about what I would want if I were the patient in that very situation. It is hard to fault our motives and decision-making if we did what we would have wanted for our own eye.

> We surgeons go into every cataract surgery knowing that on rare occasions, despite our best efforts, the capsule or its supporting fibers called "zonules" may split during the fragmenting and removal of the cataract. In your case, the capsule split, but I was able to remove the majority of the cataract. When the capsule splits, what type of lens implant to use and how best to secure it into position become difficult decisions. Even though the eye needs an artificial lens in order to see properly, it doesn't necessarily have to be placed at the same time as the cataract surgery. We can also return to the operating room in a month or so to place the lens implant after the eye has healed from the original cataract surgery and after we have more of an opportunity to evaluate which lens implant design is best to use based on the amount of remaining capsule in your eye.

> While facing this decision during surgery, and knowing that you'd be very disappointed to need a second operation, I'll admit that I was tempted to just place a lens implant into your eye. However, this is an important decision and I didn't want

to rush into placing a type of lens implant that I might later regret. After considering what I would want done if I were the patient, I decided that I would want the surgeon to postpone the lens implant placement until the eye was more healed and the optimal type of lens to use became clearer.

Another conversation option is the following.

Because some of the lens implant options require special skill and expertise, I would like to refer you to someone with greater experience in this type of situation. Nothing needs to be done immediately; in fact, it is better to let the eye heal further and then to reassess the anatomy before any surgical plan is decided. In the meantime, you will be very blurry. While this is very inconvenient, it is quite expected. This blur will not determine or affect your final outcome. I know that this must be surprising and disappointing for you. I am very sorry for the stress that this is causing and that you are going to have the inconvenience of a second procedure. However, I am pleased that I succeeded in completing the rest of the surgery and I believe that your prognosis is still excellent. As difficult as it is, we all will just need to be patient.

THE DROPPED NUCLEUS

Robert H. Osher, MD and David F. Chang, MD

From Robert H. Osher, MD

In my situation, I have a fully staffed retinal team available and there is almost always at least one who is operating in a nearby room. Over 40 years, I have dropped 7 nuclei, and these occurred most often when there was either a brunescent, mature cataract or a posterior polar cataract. Unless the nucleus is dangling within my reach and amenable to a PAL (posterior-assisted levitation) maneuver, I proceed to clean up the cortex and any vitreous in the anterior segment, while resisting the temptation to go after this seductive nucleus. I will either put a lens in the torn capsular bag or use one of the optic captures. Fortunately, this is a very rare event, but I have never had a patient angry because I sent them from Room 5 to Room 1 (where one of the retina surgeons is working) for an "adjustment" following an honest and reassuring explanation.

> I wish I could tell you that everything went perfect in the operating room today, but it didn't. We typically break the cataract up into tiny fragments and remove it through a small incision in the front of the eye. Your cataract went just the opposite way and dropped backwards into the back of the eye. Although this is a well-known complication, no surgeon likes to see this happen for a number of reasons. First, we want every operation to be perfect, and if doesn't go perfect, we have to manage the complication the best we can. Second, we have to ask our retinal colleagues who specialize in back-of-the-eye problems to help us remove the cataract because cataract surgeons typically work in the front of the eye, which is a whole different neighborhood. This extra effort is necessary, if we expect to achieve an excellent outcome... which we do. I apologize for the detour we are going to have to take, and I'll do everything I can to introduce you to an excellent retinal specialist who will help us reach our goal of improving your vision by removing the remaining piece.

From David F. Chang, MD

For a retained nucleus, I usually try to have the patient seen by the retina specialist within 1 to 2 days. If there is an intervening weekend or wait of a few days, I would check the patient in the interim to check the IOP.

> We surgeons go into every cataract surgery knowing that on rare occasions, despite our best efforts, the capsule may split during the fragmenting and removal of the cataract. This can allow one of the smaller pieces to slip back through this split in the capsule, and drift toward the back of the eyeball. This happened as I was removing your cataract. Even though the eyeball is small, for the purpose of surgery we divide the inside of the eyeball into 2 halves—the front and the back halves. Cataract, cornea, and glaucoma surgeries are all done in the front half. Surgery done for the retina or the vitreous gel within the eye are done in the back half. Retina surgeons operate within the back half of the eye and they use different incisions, different instruments, and different viewing systems than we use in the front half of the eye. Even though a dozen different eye surgeons operate at this surgery center, we are all "front-of-the-eye" surgeons; retina surgeons operate at a different center because of the different equipment that they need.

> When one of the cataract fragments slips to the back half of the eye, it is always safer to have the retina surgeon remove it, even though this requires a second operation. Knowing that this is inconvenient for patients, it is always tempting for cataract surgeons to try to fish out that small piece of the cataract. However, because our view into the back half isn't very good, this can result in serious accidental damage to the retina. So even though it was tempting to try to fish for that little piece of lens, I decided that if this were my eye, it would be better and safer to have a retina specialist do a second operation to remove it in a week or so from now.

> Fortunately, I was able to complete the rest of the operation and to insert the artificial lens in a good position. I'm actually very pleased with how well the remainder of the surgery went under the circumstances. So the plan now will be to have you see one of the best retina surgeons in the area, who can then

remove that small fragment of the cataract in the next week or so. It is still an outpatient operation and it is still performed through very tiny incisions.

I know that this must be very disappointing and unpleasant for you. Putting myself in your shoes, I can imagine how worried and surprised you must be. I am very sorry for the stress that this is causing and that you are going to have the inconvenience of a second procedure. However, I am pleased that I succeeded in completing the rest of the operation, and I believe that your prognosis is still excellent. Naturally, it will be very blurry in the beginning and you'll see some large floaters at first. This blur doesn't determine or affect your final outcome. I'm optimistic that you'll probably see quite well in 4 to 6 weeks, or possibly sooner. We're going to arrange the appointment with the retina specialist, who will be able to give you more information about the second procedure. I'll phone you after that consultation to see if you have any additional questions that didn't come up today.

CAN'T PLACE MICROINVASIVE GLAUCOMA SURGERY DEVICE

Jack S. Parker, MD, PhD

This is a potentially embarrassing situation, because you've likely taken special time out of your normal cataract conversation to convince the patient why they should have this extra procedure and now you have to return and explain why you couldn't do it.

My best tip for how to negotiate this conversation relates to avoiding it. After the IOL is implanted, intracameral instillation of Trypan blue directed into the nasal angle selectively stains the pigmented TM bright blue and helps differentiate the angle structures and provides an aiming target or landmark for MIGs procedures. This improves visualization of the relevant anatomy, and as a result this conversation may become less frequent. Nevertheless, what I say on those occasions is the following.

> The cataract surgery went perfectly. At the end of the surgery, we tried to place that extra little glaucoma device that we talked about, but we discovered that our view into that part of the eye was not good enough to do it safely. So, we decided just to stop while we were ahead and not put the thing in, after all (Figure 2-3). But, I'm confident you're going to do great, that both your vision and your pressure are going to be improved.

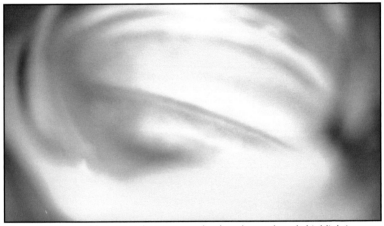

Figure 2-3. Trypan blue stains the pigmented trabecular meshwork, highlighting your target. (Reprinted with permission from Parker JS, Parker A, Parker JS. Trypan blue-assisted microinvasive glaucoma surgery. *J Cataract Refract Surg.* 2017;43:1613.)

THE PATIENT WITH A BRUISE

Robert H. Osher, MD

When I walk out to visit the patient after surgery, I always apologize for any bruising on the lids. If the bruise is noticed on the day after surgery, I'll reassure the patient, and then ask if the husband (or wife) did this. (They always laugh). Then I tell the patient that it matches the rose or carnation we give every patient for the past 4 decades. Reassurance with a little humor is usually well received by the patient.

In the recovery room this is the usual conversation.

> Mr. or Ms. _____, I see that you have an impressive bruise on your skin. It looks like we used boxing gloves instead of surgery gloves! This is from the anesthetic that the anesthesia team gave you to numb your eye—so, I am innocent! *[and I wink].* I'm sorry you have a bruise, but it will not cause any problem and will go away like any other bruise after a few days.

WHAT I SAY TO THE PATIENT IMMEDIATELY AFTER ROUTINE SURGERY

Robert H. Osher, MD

I realize it is not very efficient, but at the stage I am at currently in my career, maximizing the number of surgeries is not important to me. I prefer that each surgery—in fact, each patient encounter, preparation and planning, operation, and the postoperative experience—is as good as I can possibly provide to every patient. After the patient is taken to their recovery room and is reunited with their family who has watched the surgery, I will enter the room, introduce myself again (since my mask is on), and shake hands with the family member saying that I hope he or she enjoyed watching. I will walk to the opposite side of the stretcher so that I can address both the patient and the family "eye-to-eye." I'll begin by saying the following.

> Mr. or Mrs. _____, the cataract surgery went very well, and I am very pleased. Judy is one of our best nurses; she will go over everything today and I will repeat the instructions tomorrow, giving you a double dose of instructions just in case your memory is like mine.

Here I will wink. If the patient has received a block, I will go on to say the following.

> You are going to notice some double vision for a few hours because the eyes cannot work together until the anesthetic has disappeared in a few hours.

To demonstrate how the eyes work together, I move my 2 index fingers in unison back and forth. I may close the lid with a steri-strip to eliminate the diplopia, also protecting the cornea.

> Because we don't use sutures anymore and simply swell the small incisions closed, your vision may be blurry for a few days until the swelling goes down and then your vision will improve.

To explain the relationship between the swelling and the vision, I make a gesture with my thumb down, then I switch my thumb upward. This goes back to the basic philosophy of preparing the patient for the worst, so he or she will be pleasantly surprised on the first postoperative day.

Now I look at the family member and say the following.

> I want you to spoil and pamper my patient—I did my best and now it's your turn.

I look back at the patient and put my hand on his or her shoulder.

> I'm going to turn you over to Judy's good hands and I'm going to take mine back to work. Judy will give you my cell phone number in case you have any questions or concerns, and I'll look forward to seeing you tomorrow.

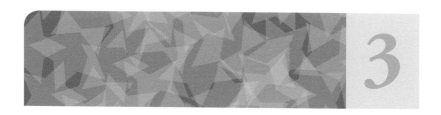

POSTOPERATIVE
CONVERSATIONS

Osher RH, Parker JS.
*What I Say: Conversations That Improve the
Physician-Patient Relationship (pp 71-103).*
© 2019 Taylor & Francis Group.

71

WHAT I SAY TO THE PATIENT ON THE FIRST POSTOPERATIVE DAY

Robert H. Osher, MD

After I review the recorded vision, confrontation visual field, IOP, and examine the eye with the slit lamp, I have this conversation

> Let me briefly review your instructions again. First, wear your eye shield for a few nights when you are sleeping so you don't accidentally rub your eye. Second, no heavy lifting for a couple of weeks. Normal lifting is okay, but if it's heavy let the boss do it.

Here I point to the husband, wife, or other family member.

> Third, follow your little instruction sheet for your drops—you can't possibly go wrong by filling in the little circles. Fourth, you'll come back for a routine 3-week visit, and you will be seen up here by one of my partners while I am operating up a storm downstairs in surgery. But if you need me, you've got my cell phone number. Fifth, the IOL has a built-in sunglass. You can still wear your sunglasses, but if you don't you're still protected from harmful UV sunlight. Sixth, my team will talk to you about your need for glasses when we give you your next appointment. Lastly, you can have the cataract in your other eye scheduled whenever you wish.

> Here's a little flower from our team. It's our way of saying thank you for being a great patient yesterday.

If the eye is a little red, I say that the rose (woman) or the carnation (man) matches the eye, and wink (Figure 3-1). Over 40 years, I think I've given out acres of flowers! At this point, my scheduling person has just walked into the room in response to my pressing a buzzer and I shake a few hands before gracefully exiting.

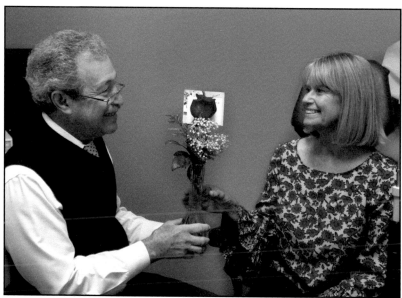

Figure 3-1. Patients appreciate a little extra kindness.

Bonus: Postoperative
Instructions and Medication Sheet

Robert H. Osher, MD

We print the following pages together on a single, 2-sided sheet (Figures 3-2 and 3-3) for all our cataract surgery patients and ask them to bring it with them to all their postoperative visits. This significantly reduces patient confusion and enhances (and effectively tracks!) compliance with topical medications.

		Day 1	Day 2	Day 3	Day 4	Day 5	Day 6	Day 7
Week 1	VIGAMOX	OOOO	OOOO	OOOO	OOOO	STOP		
	DUREZOL	OOOO	OOOO	OOOO	OOOO	OOOO	OOOO	OOOO
Week 2	DUREZOL	OO	OO	OO	OO	OO	OO	OO
Week 3	ILEVRO	O	O	O	O	O	O	O
Week 4	ILEVRO	O	O	O	O	O	O	O
Week 5	ILEVRO	O	O	O	O	O	O	O
Week 6	ILEVRO	O	O	O	O	O	O	O

CEI — CINCINNATI EYE INSTITUTE — Robert H. Osher, M.D. Eye Drop Schedule

*Keep your eye gently closed after drop is instilled and wait 5 minutes between drops

Figure 3-2. Postoperative drop regimen.

CEI
CINCINNATI EYE INSTITUTE

Robert H. Osher, MD
Blue Ash Office:
Cell:

GENERAL POST-OPERATIVE INSTRUCTIONS

"DO's"

- ☐ Tape your protective shield over your eye at bedtime or naptime to prevent accidentally rubbing or bumping your eye. Wear the shield as directed by your surgeon.
- ☐ The post-operative eye drops are VERY IMPORTANT. Use them as directed on your drop schedule.
- ☐ Always bring your post-operative bag with all of your drops and instruction sheet to all of your visits.
- ☐ Keep the area around your eye clean.
- ☐ You may return to work any time, provided your job does not require heavy lifting or straining. If your job requires exertion, please discuss with your doctor.
- ☐ You may sleep in any position; just remember to wear your shield according to your surgeon's instructions.

"DO NOTS"

- ☐ Do not lift anything over 25 lbs. for the first week. No more than 50 lbs. for the first month after surgery.
- ☐ Do not rub your eye. This is the worst thing you can do while it's healing.
- ☐ Do not wash your hair the first 24 hours after surgery.
- ☐ Do not use soap around your eye for the first 2-3 days. Just gently cleanse the lids with a clean face cloth moistened with warm water.
- ☐ Do not wear makeup for 4 days.

WHAT TO EXPECT AND WATCH FOR:

- ☐ You may experience temporary fluttering, shimmering, or floaters (black or grey specks) in your post-operative eye, but these should disappear. You should have no pain after surgery.
- ☐ Your eye may feel slightly irritated or scratchy and you may take two Tylenol to relieve this.
- ☐ Your eye may appear red or bloodshot. This will gradually lessen as your eye heals.

CALL THE OFFICE IMMEDIATELY SHOULD YOU EXPERIENCE ANY OF THE FOLLOWING:

- ☐ Sudden decrease in vision.
- ☐ Increase in pain.
- ☐ Shower of new floaters.
- ☐ Veil across vision, like a curtain in front of your eye.
- ☐ Flashes of light.

TIME FRAME FOR SOME COMMON ACTIVITIES:

- ☐ **Golf:** Putting and chipping allowed after one week. Driving the golf ball allowed after two weeks (three weeks after a toric lens). Do not carry your bag for three weeks.
- ☐ **Exercise:** Walking right away. Running/jogging in three weeks.
- ☐ **Driving:** This will depend on your post-operative vision. Discuss with your doctor.

Figure 3-3. Instructions for patients following surgery.

ONE DAY POSTOPERATIVE: MY VISION IS WORSE THAN BEFORE SURGERY!

Robert H. Osher, MD

Mr. or Mrs. _____, remember yesterday after surgery when I explained that we do not use stitches anymore, rather we deliberately swell the small incision closed. I asked you to be patient because your vision would be blurred for a few days following surgery until the normal swelling has resolved. Give it a few days for your vision to clear, and I'm confident that we're going to have an excellent result.

DYSPHOTOPSIAS

Robert H. Osher, MD

While I have rarely had to exchange a lens for either positive or negative dysphotopsia, I have certainly spent considerable time explaining the temporal crescent-shaped shadow to many patients. In fact, I conducted a study questioning 250 consecutive patients on the first postoperative day and then again after the postoperative period to understand the incidence of this puzzling symptom. You would be surprised how common it is immediately after surgery, yet it is almost always gone after the eye has healed. I hypothesized that the transient temporal crescent (not the permanent symptom) is due to the localized swelling of the temporal incision and I developed a technique at the slit lamp to show what the patient is seeing. If the illuminator is held in your outside hand, and you rotate it back and forth passing light through the incision edge, you can see a shadow of a straight line on the iris when the light is perpendicular, and it curves into a crescent as the illuminator is rotated temporally casting a crescent-shaped shadow near the pupil. It is very dramatic. So, when the patient tells me that they see this in the early postoperative period, here is what I say.

> Please don't worry about that shadow you see off to the side because it is very commonly noticed right after surgery. It's probably due to the mild swelling of the little incision, and will disappear as the eye is healing. Rarely, somebody can see the curved edge of their implant just like I can see the edge of my glasses, but it's absolutely nothing to worry about. You're going to have an excellent result.

By reassuring the patient, I cannot recall having to either exchange or piggyback one of my own patients, although I have performed this procedure for several referred patients. I am certain that this common complaint began when the temporal incision became popular. Yet, I also understand that a rare patient can have permanent negative dysphotopsia related to the optics of the lens edge; that requires a lengthier discussion which is beyond the scope of this chapter.

WHEN THE PATIENT COMPLAINS ABOUT THE HIGH COST OF POSTOPERATIVE DROPS

Robert H. Osher, MD

We used to give out tons of samples, but our supply has been severely reduced by the companies. Moreover, I understand the lengthy and costly process of getting a drug through the FDA, so every company has a right to make a reasonable return on their investment. Yet, I really sympathize with the patients who stand little chance of winning this economic battle given the strong pharmaceutical lobby.

> Mr. or Mrs. _____, I couldn't agree more with you. In fact, if you add up the cost of the antibiotic, the steroid, and the NSAID, you're actually paying more for the drops than I get paid by Medicare to perform the operation! I always prescribe the drops that I think are the best for you, but we would be happy to substitute a generic medication if you prefer. But I hope you will be having cataract surgery only once in your right or left eye, and I would personally prefer to have the most protective drops for this once-in-a-lifetime special occasion.

POSTERIOR CAPSULAR OPACIFICATION

Robert H. Osher, MD

Mr. or Mrs. _____, with this microscope I can see why your vision has become a bit cloudy. You may remember that the cataract was surrounded by a very thin cellophane-like membrane that we polished and left in the eye to hold the IOL. We call this the capsule, and it shrinks down to lock the lens in place. In some patients, this clear membrane becomes a little cloudy over time, like wax paper, and the vision becomes a little blurred. We no longer need the center portion of this capsule once the lens implant becomes a part of the eye. We used to take the patient back to surgery and perform a second operation on what we called a "secondary cataract." Fortunately, we no longer have to do this, and instead simply press a button to generate a laser beam that quickly and harmlessly evaporates the capsule. It is painless and it only takes a couple of minutes to perform. I believe it will clear up your vision. So, if you'd like to have this done, my assistant will review the details (benefits and risks) and have you sign a consent form, so we can help you recover clear vision ASAP.

The conversation is similar if the patient notes light streaks due to parallel striate in the posterior capsule.

REFRACTIVE SURPRISE

Robert H. Osher, MD

If the patient has received a premium IOL, we would be more likely to encourage either a lens exchange or refer the patient to our refractive team for a laser "touch-up." Piggybacking a secondary lens is seldom used in our practice and would require extenuating circumstances, like a longstanding "fibrosed" capsular bag in an eye with a spacious posterior chamber, an eye with a large radial tear in the anterior capsule, or post-YAG laser capsulotomy. I personally prefer an IOL exchange or corneal laser enhancement.

> Mr. or Mrs. _____, I understand that you are disappointed because your vision is still not crystal clear after surgery. We always try to improve the vision by 2 ways whenever we operate. The first way is by removing the cataract that caused your blurred vision. The second way is to give you an implant that will reduce your nearsightedness, farsightedness, or astigmatism. We select this implant by complex formulas that depend upon the length of the eye, the curvature of the cornea, and exactly where the implant sits inside the eye after it has healed. We can measure the length of the eye to a hundredth of a millimeter and the cornea to a hundredth of a diopter. But everybody heals differently, and it is impossible to know exactly where the lens will seal into place. We do our best to select the perfect lens, but not every lens prescription is manufactured so we are always erring up or down. No matter how hard we try, we are still unable to make every patient see perfectly clear without glasses.
>
> Occasionally, the cataract surgeon will have to exchange the lens. Of course, a simple pair of glasses or contact lenses will usually bring the vision into clear focus, but every cataract surgeon wants to meet the expectations of his or her patients. And even if the surgery is perfect, the art of selecting exactly the right lens is still far from perfect. So in a case like your's, we should discuss the option of returning to the operating room where we can exchange the lens, or sending you to our refractive team for a laser adjustment. I'm optimistic that we can get closer to our goal of achieving clear vision with less dependence on glasses.

WHEN A LASER "TOUCH-UP" IS NECESSARY AFTER CATARACT SURGERY

Richard L. Lindstrom, MD

Author's note from Robert H. Osher, MD: I met Dick Lindstrom, MD nearly 40 years ago, and we immediately became fast friends. There is no ophthalmologist who has better communication skills than Dick, which has been a primary reason that he has built one of the most successful mega-practices, made countless contributions to the industry, and remains one of the most sought-after lecturers on the planet.

Postoperative enhancements are a part of modern cataract surgery, whether a standard IOL or so-called "premium IOL" is selected. My conversation with the patient starts at the initial visit. I tell them the following.

> The best visual outcomes usually require 3 steps. First, a meticulous and well-planned cataract surgery. Second, 1 or 2 laser enhancement treatments in the office to fine-tune the visual outcome. And third, up to a year of neuroadaptation to adjust to your new vision.

If I do not need steps 2 and 3, everyone is happy, and I am a hero. I have found that patients and their families remember better when they hear things multiple times, so I usually say it 2 or 3 times in different ways. I might say the following at a second time.

> So we will start with quality surgery, and we are very experienced in cataract surgery and have the best equipment and a great team. Then you may benefit from 1 or 2 office-based laser enhancements to achieve the best vision. And remember, it will take a while for you to adapt to your new vision.

If I am not dealing with an especially demanding, dysfunctional, distressed, or demented patient or family, the discussion I have is relatively short. When needed, I take as much time as necessary. With difficult or complex cases, I do not hesitate to stop the discussion and go see another patient, allowing the patient time to talk with their family and my scribe/

patient counselor, before I return again for more conversation. In rare cases, I will recommend another visit with me or a second opinion. At the end of the consultation, I always ask if the patient or family has any questions, thank them for coming, and (if they are happy) encourage them to refer their friends and family to our practice. On the way up and out of the room, I may remind them a third time that we start with quality surgery, then perform laser enhancements as needed, and finally allow them adequate time to adapt to their new vision. I often reassure them that we perform this surgery frequently, are good at it, and will guide them through the process. I use EMR (electronic medical records) and have a scribe/patient counselor who remains in the room when I leave and answers any further questions and reaffirms my message. Then the patient is transferred to a surgery councilor/scheduler who again answers questions, reaffirms the message, and schedules the surgery. Finally, patients and their families are given a number to call with any further questions. Our practice is also working hard to strengthen our patient education before they are seen by distributing written educational materials, strengthening our website, and utilizing programs like MD Backline and Checked Up.

In the postoperative period, especially with patients in the premium channel, I am very aggressive with YAG laser and excimer laser refractive enhancements. I find that even very mild capsular opacity and residual refractive error, especially astigmatism, can significantly impact quality of vision with a toric or diffractive optic premium IOL; resulting in reduced patient satisfaction. I like to perform YAG laser capsulotomy prior to excimer laser refractive enhancements in most cases, as I have found the manifest refraction often changes slightly and at a minimum the refraction is more accurate with the capsule open. I will regularly say the following to a patient.

> Your vision is good, but I can make it even better with 2 low-risk office laser treatments, and I encourage you to have them done.

I prefer to use "treatments" rather than surgical procedures, and will often describe this process as "enhancing" and "fine-tuning" or "refining" the outcome. If the patient choses to proceed, I then discuss in more detail the process, potential benefits and risks, and of course the alternatives—which include doing nothing or wearing glasses or (rarely) contact lenses. For the patient who is a cash pay participant in our premium channel option, there is no charge for these laser enhancements.

For patients who did not opt for our cash pay premium channel, my indications for YAG laser capsulotomy are similar to that for cataract surgery itself, and we charge and bill insurance as appropriate. I do find that many patients who did not originally select the premium channel are often interested after surgery in enhancing their no-glasses visual performance, especially at distance; and I do offer them excimer laser refractive enhancements at a reduced charge. The ultimate goal is a happy patient who will speak positively to friends and family about me and our practice and generate word of mouth referrals.

I should mention that while I am more aggressive than many in my refractive cataract surgery patients with both YAG laser and excimer laser refractive enhancements, I am extremely conservative in regard to IOL exchange. I cannot recall performing an IOL exchange on one of my own premium IOL patients. I have found that unless a multifocal IOL is placed in a patient with reduced contrast sensitivity for other reasons (such as corneal pathology including radial keratotomy, prior laser corneal refractive surgery with significant induced higher order aberrations, Fuch's dystrophy, Salzmans, epithelial basement membrane dystrophy or EBMD, severe dry eye and the like, or macular or optic nerve pathology), they nearly always neuro adapt if given enough time. This is why I like to tell all patients that it can take up to a year and occasionally more to fully adapt to their new vision. In my experience, the patient who is initially unhappy with their outcome nearly always responds to aggressive therapy for their ocular surface, laser enhancement, and (if possible) treatment of any corneal or retinal pathology. In conclusion, for me it is informing the patient that a successful outcome usually requires 3 steps: meticulous surgery, one or more laser enhancements to enhance the visual outcome, and tincture of time to neuro adapt to their new vision.

THE UNHAPPY PATIENT DESPITE A GOOD RESULT

Robert H. Osher, MD

These patients can be really tough, because perception is reality. Through the eyes of a surgeon, it is frustrating when the patient can't seem to appreciate your beautiful work. Yet, *it is essential that the physician resist the temptation to berate the patient for his inaccurate opinion* that his or her vision is no better after surgery than it was before surgery. The following is what I say.

> Mr. or Mrs. _____, I understand that you may have expected a miracle, but I am not a miracle worker. But I am a very detailed record keeper and here is what your vision was before surgery.

At this point I will isolate the preoperative Snellen line to demonstrate the preoperative acuity.

> Not only that, our testing in bright lights with glare indicated that your vision was legally blind.

I'll put up the big E while showing them their acuity on the medical record. If the other eye has a cataract, I will then request that they cross-cover one eye at a time and compare. If the patient is a hyperope or myope in the unoperated eye, this is especially impressive as they are comparing their uncorrected vision.

> I'm sure you can see how much your vision has improved!

Now if you missed your refractive target, that's an entirely different story, which is the reason that I always tell patients that they may need a thin pair of glasses after surgery. If the patient is left with unexpected low myopia, I will show them that their vision is perfectly clear up close. A little hyperopic error is managed by showing them a real-time video of their anterior segment and commenting that the eye looks "unoperated." I like to remind the patient of the following.

> Even a perfect operation may leave a little nearsightedness, farsightedness, or astigmatism because everyone heals differently.

Again, it's always better to under-promise and over-deliver. By taking the time to compare the unaided vision in one eye to the other and demonstrating the preoperative and postoperative vision Snellen lines, the patient can be educated to recognize the improvement for which he or she will probably be grateful.

THE UNHAPPY MULTIFOCAL PATIENT

Richard J. Mackool, MD and Robert J. Cionni, MD

Author's note from Robert H. Osher, MD: Dick Mackool, MD is an intrepid master cataract surgeon with more than 40 years of experience in handling complex cases referred from around the world. The more challenging the patient, the more he seems to relish the opportunity to intervene in the patient's visual behalf.

Sometimes it's not what you tell them after the surgery, it's what information you gave them before the surgery that is most important.

The postoperative discussion is greatly simplified if the possible outcomes of multifocal IOL implantation were discussed, or better yet given to the patient in an easy to read handout, before the preoperative consultation. The risk of problems such as glare or halo, inadequate intermediate and/or near vision, etc., as well as the potential remedies including IOL explantation should absolutely be presented at that time. Relevant questions should be answered during a leisurely and non-stressful preoperative conversation. If this has not been done and a multifocal IOL-related issue develops, fasten your seatbelt because you're in for a rough ride. In the latter situation, options include: 1) apologies; 2) refunding payments; 3) calling your attorney; 4) all of the above.

Author's note from Robert H. Osher, MD: Upon finishing his cataract fellowship at CEI, Bob Cionni, MD became a tour de force in the field of cataract surgery. For his many innovations, he was honored in 2018 as the Kelman Lecturer at the AAO.

Let me begin by saying that the situation of achieving a perfect refractive result and still having an unhappy multifocal IOL patient is much less common than it was it the past. I credit this trend to better technology, a better understanding of who will do well with a multifocal IOL, and more emphasis on educating our patients preoperatively about realistic expectations. Still, we will occasionally see a perfect or near-perfect refractive result and a disappointed patient. How one handles this situation is vitally important to whether the patient leaves your office happy with the care they received or prepared to tell all their friends to never consider going to your practice for care. All of us went into the practice of ophthalmology to help patients see better. When we don't please our patients, it is deeply disturbing to us as well.

How we turn this unhappy situation into one that results in a satisfied patient depends on what you say to your patient and what you do for your patient. This begins before surgery by painting realistic expectations. Still, you will find an occasional patient that, despite doing your best to educate preoperatively, their expectations exceeded their result. I see this most frequently with the low to moderate myope who reads without glasses preoperatively, but needs cataract surgery to improve their distance vision. It is imperative to emphasize to this patient before surgery that their reading vision will never be as good as it was in the past without glasses with a multifocal IOL, and if they expect such a result then they are not a good candidate. It is amazing how many patients don't truly listen to that advice, so definitely document that conversation. In this situation, I always offer the patient an IOL exchange, but provide a detailed explanation of the benefits, risks, and limitations of the results. For example, if they still want distance vision without glasses then they will still need readers, as they already do now.

Let's go through an example of what I would say to this patient who typically is happy with their distance vision, but not their near vision. Please note that how you talk to your patient, including both verbal and nonverbal cues, is extremely important. Yes, you are as frustrated as the patient. Yet in this situation, the surgeon needs to set their feelings and judgments aside and manage the patient with complete empathy. Put yourself in their shoes or imagine that the patient is your mother… I often use this trick to put myself in the correct mindset to best handle the situation.

> Mr. Smith, I understand that you are happy with your driving vision, but you're frustrated with the quality of your near vision. Let me examine your eyes to see if there is anything I can find to explain your frustration.

I have been amazed how a moderate amount of PC wrinkling can disturb near vision with a multifocal IOL. However, in this example, either the capsule is pristine or a YAG capsulotomy has already been performed and everything else is normal. After the exam I sit back in a relaxed position and say the following.

> Well, everything looks perfect Mr. Smith. Do me a favor and read as low as you can on this reading card.

The patient reads the J1 line, but with a bit of a struggle.

> I'm going to put a pair of glasses on you that simulates what you would be able to read up close had we put a standard IOL in instead of the multifocal IOL.

The patient states, "I can't read anything". I then say this.

> Unfortunately, that is what your vision would be up close without readers had we put a standard IOL in… so you now understand that the multifocal IOL is providing you some ability to read without glasses. Yet, I know that your reading vision is not as crisp as you would like it to be. When you need to see more crisply up close, such as when you are reading a small print novel, you can always put on readers to magnify and sharpen your near vision. But, in time you will likely be doing so less and less as you get used to the multifocal IOL.

You may need to show the patient your documented preoperative discussion at this point. I then go on to say the following.

> However, if you want, I can exchange this IOL for a standard IOL and aim for either near or distance vision, but if I do so you will always need glasses for one of these distances. If you chose to do this, we will fully refund the additional money you paid for your multifocal IOL.

Yes…it is not about the money!!! Do not hesitate to fully refund the patient's out of pocket paid for the multifocal IOLs. They need to know that your motivation is purely about making them happy with their vision!

Typically, the patient decides to keep the multifocal IOL. Yet, the situation is not over as the patient is still not thrilled. So, this is the time when you need to encourage the patient to come back for further follow up.

> Mr. Smith, I want to see you back in a couple months to see make certain your near vision is improving. Yet, if at any time, you decide you want to have the multifocal IOLs removed, I will be happy to do so. However, if you decide to have the IOLs exchanged and aim for distance vision without glasses, then I really believe an IOL exchange will not provide you with any real benefit. Your distance vision will likely remain the same, yet you will definitely eliminate any ability to read without

glasses, while you have some reading ability without glasses now.

Make certain that each conversation is fully documented, as we all know that patients tend not to remember the details of everything said during an office visit.

Seeing and talking to these patients is not the most enjoyable part of our day. But at these times it is important to run towards the patient and not away, in order to maintain a good relationship. If you treat each patient as you would a family member, this is much easier to do. If you handle these situations empathetically, both you and the patient will feel better.

When the Patient Asks for a Second Opinion

Robert H. Osher, MD

It is essential to not be offended when a patient requests a second opinion. Even minimal reluctance by the treating ophthalmologist can be interpreted as defensive behavior. The best way to maintain a strong patient-physician relationship is to show genuine concern and willingness to help the patient. It is beneficial to offer the names of other competent ophthalmologists, rather than to allow the patient to select by potluck. I am aware of a number of lawsuits that were initiated by the comments of an unfriendly competitor who tried to elevate his stature by diminishing that of the treating ophthalmologist. If the patient is concerned for any reason, it's always best to go "above and beyond" in offering support and attention.

> Mr. or Mrs. _____, I understand your concern, and I agree that second opinions are sometimes very helpful. But the value of the opinion will depend upon the expertise of the doctor that you see. I can offer you several names of very competent ophthalmologists who will give you an honest and knowledgeable second opinion. Sometimes getting in to see these experts can be difficult, and my staff would be happy to help you schedule an appointment if you wish. I always welcome another opinion, if there is any additional possibility of helping you get the best result.

WHEN THE PATIENT COMES TO SEE YOU FOR A SECOND OPINION
Warren E. Hill, MD, FACS

Author's note from Robert H. Osher, MD: Warren Hill, MD, FACS has not only mastered IOL selection, but he has also mastered the art of communication. His lectures are before standing-room only crowds in the United States and abroad, who attend to pay tribute to his decades of providing help to both patients and colleagues.

Before seeing the patient, I have my staff do the usual measurements that I would do prior to cataract surgery. This includes axial measurements and autokeratometry, a topographic axial curvature map, an assessment of the posterior cornea, and a macular optical coherence tomography (OCT). This also serves as a quick check to make sure that the refractive surprise was not due to something like overlooking prior refractive surgery, undiagnosed keratoconus, elevated higher order aberrations, or the presence of CME. If available, I also check prior records to see what IOL was implanted and the target spherical equivalent. With all of this in hand I enter the examination room, introduce myself, and begin the discussion after a brief examination at the slit lamp to confirm that the IOL is completely within the capsular bag and has good anterior capsule overlap.

> My staff tells me that the outcome of your cataract surgery ended up different than expected.

Here I have the patient tell me how it was different. This is very important, as one common complaint is that no one may have listened to them in a way that was meaningful. If they had, we probably would not be having this conversation.

> When doing cataract surgery, we replace the natural lens of the eye with an artificial one. These are the measurements that we use to determine the power of this artificial lens. In addition, there are the formulas that we use to estimate the power of this artificial lens. By estimate, what I mean to say is that there is currently no way to exactly calculate the power of this artificial lens. Most of the time we get this right, but not always.

One important aspect of selecting this lens power is based on something that can only be estimated and not calculated.

I refer to the effective lens position.

Sometimes, when the estimation of the formula does not exactly match the individual anatomy of the eye, we get an outcome that's different than anticipated. For most lens powers, all it takes is a 0.5 mm mis-estimation of this critical value for a 1.00 D error in the intraocular lens power.

I then ask the patient to hold their fingers 0.5 mm apart and at the same time pick a 1.00 D lens from a loose lens set.

A 1.00 mm mis-estimation is a 2.00 D error.

I will pick that lens from a loose lens set and show it to them.

The higher the power of the lens, the more critical this value becomes. We repeated your measurements and got basically the same numbers. In your case, the assumptions of the various formulas we commonly use did not appear to match the anatomy of your eye.

The good news is that we can go back and exchange the lens you presently have for one of a different power. This calculation is not an estimation and is far more accurate, as we already know the power and the position of the lens that was implanted. I expect that after a lens exchange there is a good chance that we will get the desired result in terms of the refractive outcome.

DISLOCATED OR WRONG POWER INTRAOCULAR LENS

Robert H. Osher, MD

I do not have a routine patter for this complication; I hope no one does. These cases are exceptionally unusual and once again, honesty is the best policy. Of course, one must toss in a pinch of sincere concern and reassurance. Patients like knowing the truth and appreciate when your eyes meet theirs and when you gently touch their arm or shoulder with a pat of kindness. They can sense either your interest or disinterest as well as when you are "covering up" or being untruthful. I cast my vote for diplomatic transparency.

For the first couple of decades of my referral cataract practice, I saw a significant number of refractive surprises and decentered lenses. We did not know how to deal with postrefractive patients and we were pretty bad with both high hyperopia and extreme myopia. Fortunately, the biometry and IOL formulas improved tremendously. With respect to decentered lenses, we know more about pseudoexfoliation and have capsule-expanding devices at our disposal. We also have pupil dilating agents and devices, so we are not blindly inserting an IOL into an unknown location. Still, with high patient expectations when a premium lens is purchased, the surgeon should feel comfortable repositioning or exchanging a lens, even though this activity deals a significant blow to one's ego. I prefer an IOL exchange to laser corneal surgery if a significant refractive surprise is evident in the first month following surgery.

I remind the patient with the wrong power lens that lens selection is not a perfect science, and we use our best judgment to "guestimate" the best choice. However, lenses are made in limited powers and patients heal differently; with the slightest change in the IOL position having a marked effect on the postoperative refractive error. The postrefractive patient has been duly warned, and I explain the available options of lens exchange or corneal refractive surgery (almost never piggyback in my practice). I have also invested the time and patience with either nanophthalmos or extreme myopia, to lower their expectations of attaining clear unaided vision. Of course the surgeon should give postrefractive patients a few weeks for the refractive error to settle down, and I have seen extreme hyperopia melt away in post-RK patients. One should also understand the conversion ratio of residual refractive error to IOL power (usually 2:3), which varies with optic thickness. I will be optimistic with the patient in predicting an excellent result after an IOL exchange through a small incision to minimize induced astigmatism.

A decentered IOL requires even more explanation with a review of the zonulocapsular anatomy. I would provide an unrushed explanation and offer my recommendation. Again, I would forecast an excellent outcome. These patients deserve time, which the surgeon should willingly offer when one of these rare complications occurs.

RETAINED CHIP

Robert H. Osher, MD

Mr. or Mrs. _____, I found the reason that your healing is being delayed. There is a tiny fragment of the cataract that has found a hiding place in a remote corner in your eye that is usually invisible to us called the "angle". As you know, the small incision phacoemulsification technique uses ultrasonic energy to break the cataract into tiny fragments, which are then removed from the eye. Rarely, one of these fragments will hide either behind the iris or in the angle, 2 places that we cannot see during surgery. Sometimes these particles will dissolve on their own; but if the fragment doesn't dissolve, it can cause persistent inflammation requiring removal.

I apologize that I'm going to have to take you back to the operating room for this very brief, painless procedure, but this is the best way to get you back on the right track. Even though you had to wait when we scheduled your original surgery, I'll ask my scheduling team to prioritize this procedure and we'll have you in and out in no time.

Cystoid Macular Edema

Robert H. Osher, MD

It is always easier to explain a problem that the patient has heard about and expects rather than an unanticipated complication. For this reason, patients with a previous history of diabetic retinopathy, epiretinal membrane (ERM), vein occlusion, uveitis, or previous surgery are always told about the possibility of retinal swelling during their original evaluation. The following discussion is limited to idiopathic CME.

> Mr. or Mrs. _____, I found the cause for your blurred vision. It is a condition we call cystoid macular edema or CME, which means swelling of the retina. Although we see it quite infrequently, it used to be very common when I started my practice 40 years ago. It's hard to believe that we still don't know why the retina in the back of the eye can swell after a perfect operation in the front of the eye. It is probably a response to the normal inflammation that somehow causes the very delicate retina to swell. You notice it because your vision, which was clear after surgery, becomes more blurred. And, we can diagnose this by the way the retina appears swollen or by using very detailed photography.

> The good news is that CME almost always clears on its own, but we like to try to speed things up by bumping up your anti-inflammatory drops. Sometimes, we even send you over to the retina team where they can give you a tiny injection near the eye which is also very effective. We'll keep a close watch on your retina, which we expect to heal and your chances of achieving clear vision are excellent.

PERSISTENT
POSTOPERATIVE INFLAMMATION

Robert H. Osher, MD

If the inflammation persists, we need to perform gonioscopy to see if there is a retained nuclear chip in the angle, and the pupil will be dilated for an evaluation of where the haptics are located with respect to the capsular bag and the iris.

> When I examine your eye with the microscope, I can see evidence of residual inflammation by the presence of tiny inflammatory cells. These are the cells that the body produces to heal the eye after cataract surgery. You seem to be taking a little longer to heal, so I think we should bump up your drops. Inflammation is like a bonfire and the drops we use following surgery help to extinguish the fire. In your case, it seems like the embers are still going. So rather than using one drop a day which is a little like a squirt gun, we are going to put the fire out with more drops which act like a fire hose. We'll use _____ 4 times a day and we'll see if we have any samples. If not, I'll give you a prescription and we'll check your vision, your pressure, and look at the eye under the microscope again in several weeks. I consider this to be a temporary detour, and you should be back on track in no time with an excellent result.

DECOMPENSATED CORNEA

Jack S. Parker, MD, PhD

This is probably occurring on the heels of a complicated cataract surgery, so you may have already had some difficult conversations. As a supplement to those remarks, several months down the line I might also add the following.

> The reason that your vision is not where it needs to be is because your cornea is still swollen from the cataract surgery. We were hoping that the swelling would go away on its own, but here we are months later and it hasn't—which means we need to do something. The best thing to do is to replace the pump cells on the back of the cornea. Fortunately, that's a much easier and safer operation than the cataract surgery, and it will fix the problem and restore your vision.

At this point, I move to a discussion of endothelial transplantation, almost always Descemet membrane endothelial keratoplasty (DMEK), which is a conversation beyond the scope of this text. I should only add that although what you'd most prefer is a magic wand or a time machine that could undo whatever happened, DMEK (as opposed to Descemet's stripping automated endothelial keratoplasty or DSAEK) is the next best alternative. It offers the best visual outcomes and the fewest postoperative burdens. If at all possible, this is the surgery you should be performing for these patients, and referrals for this problem should be directed preferentially to specialists who offer it (Figure 3-4).

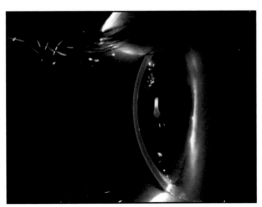

Figure 3-4. One week after DMEK with best-corrected visual acuity of 20/20.

ENDOPHTHALMITIS

Christopher D. Riemann, MD

Author's note from Robert H. Osher, MD: Chris Riemann, MD is a member of our vitreoretinal team at CEI. He is a brilliant, dynamic, and innovative surgeon whose multilingual patient discussions are direct and brutally honest—which patients always respect.

> Hi Mr. or Mrs. _____. I'm Dr. Riemann. Dr. _____ sent you in to see me urgently, is that correct?

The patient replies.

> He or she is very worried about some unexpected inflammation in your eye after your recent cataract surgery (or other procedure). When did you start having trouble?

The patient then tells their story.

> Let's take a look to see what we are dealing with here.

I will do a meticulous exam of both eyes to make sure I don't miss anything. I concentrate on what I am doing and do not talk much during the exam.

> Well, I agree with Dr. _____. You have a very, very serious problem. The inflammation in your eye is very severe. This is definitely not normal and raises the grave concern for a postoperative bacterial infection or a severe allergic-type inflammatory reaction. This inflammation represents an existential risk to your eye. That means you may not regain any vision and you may even lose your eye entirely.

Patient reacts in shock

> Yes, this is really bad. I'm very sorry. I also apologize for being so blunt, but I've always felt it very important for patients to be rapidly brought up to speed with what's going on, especially in situations like this.

Patient usually reacts with some form of gratitude.

> So, what we need to do is act quickly and decisively. I can't tell just by looking if this is an infection or just an allergic response. If it turns out that this is an allergic response, you have a pretty

good chance of doing OK and recovering at least some vision with treatment. On the other hand, if this is an infection we have to kill the bacteria right away. Bacteria double themselves every 20 minutes, so that means that every 20 minutes that we delay your treatment, there are twice as many bacteria tearing up the inside of your eye. If your inflammation is due to an infection and we delay treatment, you are guaranteed to lose your vision completely and probably lose the eye. If you're having an allergic response and we incorrectly treat it as an infection, we will have done you no harm.

You've probably noticed my staff hustling and bustling. They are getting set up for me to do an ultrasound on the eye, as well as getting everything ready for something called a tap and inject procedure that we will do right after.

The ultrasound will help me to better understand the anatomy of the back of the eye. The inflammation consists of a bunch of opaque material, or pus, that keeps you from seeing out and me from seeing in. This won't hurt at all. The ultrasound is the same thing we do to pregnant women's bellies to examine the unborn baby.

I will then perform the ultrasound and discuss the results.

The tap and inject procedure is the first step in combating this inflammation. What we're going to do for you right away is numb your eye with some anesthetic so you don't feel any pain going forward. Then we'll give you a series of 4 needles directly into the eye. The first will be an injection of more anesthetic to really numb the eye completely. Pain control is very important to me as well as you. With the second needle, I'll take a sample of fluid from the back of your eye and send it to the lab to test for bacteria. Then I'll give you 2 injections of very powerful antibiotics to kill the bacterial bugs in your eye. They'll be dead in 10 minutes. That's the good news.

Now the bad news: Even with really early diagnosis and treatment, bacterial infections sometimes don't turn out well. Your ultimate chances for recovering vision depend on how fast we get the antibiotics into your eye—as we talked about—but even more so on how aggressive of a bacterial bug we are dealing with if this is an infection. That's why I'm sending a specimen to the lab. The more common causes of these infections are usually less aggressive organisms that are everywhere on our skin. If that's what's going on here, you have a pretty good chance to get pretty decent vision back when everything is all said and done. If this is a more aggressive organism—you may have heard of "flesh eating strep," for example—then your chances of your seeing well out of this eye are much lower even with this prompt and excellent treatment. The problem is that I don't know if this is an infection at all or an allergic inflammatory reaction, let alone which bacterial bug it is. Another challenge is that only half of all bacterial infections will grow out in the lab, so there is a 50% chance we will never know if this inflammation was actually an infection or an inflammatory response.

So, all of this boils down to the unfortunate reality that I cannot honestly look you in the eye and promise you that everything will turn out OK. It may. But, even with the best possible treatment, aggressive inflammation from a bacterial infection may cause permanent visual loss. It will be many days, weeks, or even months until we'll be able to tell how this will all pan out for you. There are however some things that I can and do promise you.

1. I will be your partner and advocate throughout this process and long afterward. You and I will have a relationship until one of us dies.

2. I (or one of my partners) will always be available for you if there is a problem during your treatment.

3. I will always tell you the truth, even if it's unpleasant.

4. I will be sure to answer any questions you have as clearly and directly as possible.

5. I will fight as hard as I can for every last scrap of salvageable vision. No one will fight harder for you than me.

6. If at any point, it turns out that another doctor can do a better job than me in handling any given problem that you might develop, I promise to get that doctor involved in your care.

7. I will always utilize the team approach for your care. Dr. _____ and I will alternate checking you and will regularly communicate so we both stay up-to-date with the latest developments.

Now, let's get your treatment started. Do you have any questions?

Now I turn to the family.

Do you have any questions? Please don't hesitate to ask me anything.

The patient and or family will often ask why did this happen to him or her. They may ask if Dr. _____ did something wrong.

I wasn't in surgery, so I can't say for sure, but I honestly don't think so. These inflammatory responses, with or without infection, sometimes happen. The rate for routine cataract surgery, for example, is between 1/100 and 1/1000 depending on the source that you read. Allergies are infrequent and infections even more so; unfortunately you just drew the short straw. Another way to ask this question is to ask, "What could I have done to avoid this problem?" The answer is, you have already done it. You went to a *[insert a truthful positive attribute of the referring doctor]* cataract surgeon. He or she quickly diagnosed your problem and promptly referred you for definitive treatment and now you are here, right where you need to be. Let's get your treatment started.

Now I perform the vitreous tap and inject procedure.

Now, I know that wasn't one of your top 10 favorite recreation activities, but you took that very well. You can be proud of yourself. It's way scarier than it is painful isn't it?

The patient usually nods. The family is usually in shock at having seen what just transpired. I usually leave them in the room during the tap and inject procedure for the sake of transparency and building trust.

I turn again to the family.

> Are you guys OK? That's pretty wild isn't it? Do you see the fluid in this syringe? It should be totally clear. It's not, because the back of the eye is filled with pus. I know that's pretty gross. I'm sorry, but remember that I told you I'd always be direct.

The family agrees.

> Now let's talk about where we go from here. My scribe, _____, will now hand-courier this fluid specimen from your eye to the lab to check for bacteria. I've ordered several different tests to be done, some of which will be completed quickly and others—especially the bacterial culture result—will take up to a week to come back with results. In the meantime, we will get you started on some eye drops and we will follow you very carefully. Tomorrow's visit will be very important.

> I need to check you first thing in the morning, and I need you to not have anything to eat or drink after 12:00 midnight tonight. This is because depending on how your eye looks tomorrow, we may need to do surgery. Sometimes the tap and inject procedure is all that's needed to clear the eye up. The antibiotics kill the bacteria and the immune system absorbs and neutralizes all the associated inflammation. That's the case when the causative bacterial organism is not too aggressive. With the more aggressive organisms, like bad staph, strep, and gram negatives for example, killing the organisms causes them to rupture and spill all the chemical substances that make them so aggressive into the eye. This can make things worse. By tomorrow morning, we will have a preliminary readout on the sample that is on its way to the lab right now and I'll be able to re-examine you and tell if the dead bacteria need to be surgically removed or not.

> Do you have any questions?

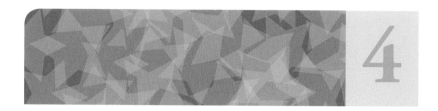

BONUS CHAPTER

WHAT I SAY TO THE REFERRING PHYSICIAN OR OPTOMETRIST

Osher RH, Parker JS.
What I Say: Conversations That Improve the
Physician–Patient Relationship (pp 105-110).
© 2019 Taylor & Francis Group.

BEFORE SURGERY, IF I AGREE WITH THE PLAN FOR CATARACT SURGERY

Robert H. Osher, MD

Throughout the 4 decades of my career, I have been aware that the success or failure of my referral cataract practice depends upon excellent communication. Not only do I send a detailed consultation letter personally written to each referral source, I call from the operating room and send a summary letter after the patient's final visit. I realize that this takes additional time, but it reflects my obsessive-compulsive personality as well as my commitment to high quality. I am certain that I could have saved legions of hours had I adapted a more streamlined approach. Yet I have no regrets about having invested the time to ensure the best communication possible to any physician or optometrist who has referred the patient for cataract consultation.

Preoperative Consultation Letter

After I complete the comprehensive history in the first paragraph, the examination findings in the second paragraph, and list the diagnoses in the third paragraph, the following paragraphs summarize my written communication to the referring doctor.

I have explained in detail the meaning and management of cataracts to Mr. or Mrs. _____, and he or she understands the elective nature of cataract surgery. Because he or she is symptomatic and the vision is no longer acceptable, I agree that cataract surgery is justified. Phacoemulsification with posterior chamber lens implantation will be scheduled under local anesthesia as an outpatient at CEI. We have spent considerable time discussing the IOL options and he or she has decided to choose a _____ IOL for distance or near.

As always, I will plan to keep you informed of Mr. or Mrs. _____'s operative and postoperative course and (if the referral source is an ophthalmologist or optometrist), I'll look forward to working with you toward this patient's visual recovery. (At this point, I will mention any other pertinent diagnosis and comment on the recommended management.) Thank you again for allowing me to evaluate your pleasant patient and for the opportunity to provide you with cataract surgical consultation.

Warmest regards,

Robert H. Osher, MD
Professor of Ophthalmology
University of Cincinnati
College of Medicine
Medical Director Emeritus
Cincinnati Eye Institute

IF I DISAGREE WITH THE INDICATION FOR CATARACT SURGERY

Robert H. Osher, MD

The following is what I tell the patient.

> Mr. or Mrs. _____, I've gone over you very thoroughly and while I agree that you have the beginning of a cataract, it's very early and there is absolutely no urgency to undergo surgery. I've never pushed a patient into the operating room, nor do I recommend surgery for patients who are still getting along fine with their vision. If your cataract progresses or if you develop bothersome symptoms, we can always schedule surgery when your vision is no longer acceptable. I'm going to send a detailed letter to Dr. _____, and I'm sure that he will appreciate our conservative approach. I'll ask him to keep an eye on your early cataract and I'm happy to see you back any time in the future.

This is what I write in the final paragraph of the consultation letter to the referring doctor.

> Dr. _____, I agree that Mr. or Mrs. _____ has an early cataract. Because her vision is still acceptable and she is content, I am going to send her back to your office so you can follow her cataract by conservative observation. I am happy to see Mr. or Mrs. _____ anytime her symptoms progress or you believe that cataract surgery is justified.
>
> Warmest regards,
>
> Robert H. Osher, MD
> Professor of Ophthalmology
> University of Cincinnati
> College of Medicine
> Medical Director Emeritus
> Cincinnati Eye Institute

IMMEDIATELY AFTER SURGERY

Robert H. Osher, MD

My scheduling assistant writes the phone number of the referring doctor's office on my surgery list, which I call the moment I finish surgery as I am signing the operating room forms.

> Good morning, this is Dr. Robert Osher from the Cincinnati Eye Institute. I'm just leaving a courtesy message for Dr. _____ as his patient, Mr. or Mrs. _____ just underwent cataract surgery. Everything went smoothly. I would appreciate if you'd share this good news with your doctor, and I hope you have a great day.

AT THE POSTOPERATIVE VISIT
Robert H. Osher, MD

Postoperative Letter After Final Visit

Dear Dr. _____,

Mr. or Mrs. _____ underwent cataract surgery with implantation of a (monofocal/toric/multifocal) IOL on (date) and the surgery went smoothly. He or she has enjoyed an uneventful postoperative course, achieving excellent vision (see attached findings). I have enjoyed caring for Mr. or Mrs. _____ and have given her the best surgical care I can render. Thank you again for allowing me to help your patient recover clear vision.

Warmest regards,

Robert H. Osher, MD
Professor of Ophthalmology
University of Cincinnati
College of Medicine
Medical Director Emeritus
Cincinnati Eye Institute

Attachment: Copy of final examination

FINANCIAL DISCLOSURES

Dr. Iqbal "Ike" K. Ahmed has not disclosed any relevant financial relationships.

Dr. Graham D. Barrett has not disclosed any relevant financial relationships.

Dr. David F. Chang has no financial or proprietary interest in the materials presented herein.

Dr. Robert J. Cionni has a consultant relationship with Alcon Laboratories.

Dr. Warren E. Hill has no financial or proprietary interest in the materials presented herein.

Dr. Anup Khatana has not disclosed any relevant financial relationships.

Dr. Douglas D. Koch is a consultant for Johnson & Johnson Vision and Carl Zeiss Meditec.

Dr. Richard L. Lindstrom is a consultant for Alcon, Bausch Health, Johnson & Johnson Vision and Carl Zeiss Meditec.

Dr. Richard J. Mackool has not disclosed any relevant financial relationships.

Dr. Samuel Masket has no financial or proprietary interest in the materials presented herein.

Dr. James M. Osher has no financial or proprietary interest in the materials presented herein.

Dr. Robert H. Osher is a consultant for the new Osher Drape design with BVI.

Dr. Jack S. Parker has no financial or proprietary interest in the materials presented herein.

Dr. Christopher D. Riemann has relationships with the following companies: Alcon, Alimera, Alimera Deutschland GmBH, Allergan, Bausch + Lomb/Valeant, BMC/Eyetube, CSTLII, Chruman Research, CVP (CEI Vision Partners), Gore, Haag Streit AG, Haag Streit Surgical, Haag Streit USA, HumanOptics AG, Iamc2, iVeena, Janssen/Johnson & Johnson Vision, Kaleidoscope Engineering, Macor Industries, MedOne, Northmark Pharmacy, NotalVision LLC, Orbit BioMedical, Reliance Industries, Salutaris MD, TrueVision, VEO, and Vortex Surgical. He has received monies for research from AGTC, Alcon, Alimera, Allergan, Arepio, Chengdu Kanghong, Clearside, Genentech/Roche, Janssen/Johnson & Johnson Vision, Lowry-MacTel Registry, Neurotech, Novartis, Ophthotec, and Regeneron.

Dr. Michael E. Snyder has performed research studies for Alcon, Johnson & Johnson Vision, and Bausch + Lomb for presbyopia-correcting IOLs.

INDEX

advanced cataract precludes visualization of fundus, 40
aggressive patients, 44
anesthesia person assigned to the room, talking to, 55
aniseikonia, 4
anticoagulant, patient on, 8
anxious patients, 43, 51–52
astigmatism, significant, 5–6. *See also* toric intraocular lenses (IOLs)

Beaver Visitec International (BVI), 51
blepharitis, 24
bruising of eye/eyelids, 67

capsular rupture. *See* posterior capsular rupture or tear
claustrophobic patients, 51–52
CME (cystoid macular edema), 34, 96
coexisting conditions
    blepharitis, 24
    cystoid macular edema, 34, 96
    diabetic retinopathy, 32
    dry eye, 25
    epiretinal membrane, 33
    epithelial basement membrane dystrophy, 26
    Fuchs' corneal dystrophy, 29–30
    glaucoma. *See* glaucoma
    keratoconus, 27–28
    macular degeneration, 31
    ocular hypertension, 35–36
complications in first eye, 41
corneal laser enhancements after cataract surgery, 80–83
cost of postoperative drops, patient complains about, 78
cystoid macular edema (CME), 34, 96

decompensated cornea, 98
Descemet membrane endothelial keratoplasty (DMEK), 98
diabetic retinopathy, 32
dislocated intraocular lens, 93–94
DMEK (Descemet membrane endothelial keratoplasty), 98
draping and claustrophobic patients, 51–52
dropped nucleus, 63–65
dry eye, 25
dysphotopsias, 77

EBMD (epithelial basement membrane dystrophy), 26
endophthalmitis, 24, 99–103
epiretinal membrane (ERM), 33
epithelial basement membrane dystrophy (EBMD), 26
equipment malfunction during surgery, 56
ERM (epiretinal membrane), 33
examination (initial), patient discussion at conclusion of, 46–48

Printed in the United States
by Baker & Taylor Publisher Services